BAS
EPIDEMIOLOGY
CONCEPTS MADE SIMPLE

DR. ANIL MISHRA

Editorial Advisor
Professor Dinesh Kumar Pal, M.D.
Head, Department of Community Medicine,
Gandhi Medical College, Bhopal

and

Dean, Faculty of Medicine,
Madhya Pradesh Medical Science University, Jabalpur

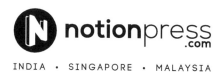

INDIA • SINGAPORE • MALAYSIA

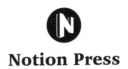

Notion Press

Old No. 38, New No. 6
McNichols Road, Chetpet
Chennai - 600 031

First Published by Notion Press 2018
Copyright © Anil Mishra 2018
All Rights Reserved.

ISBN 978-1-64249-208-8

This book has been published with all reasonable efforts taken to make the material error-free after the consent of the author. No part of this book shall be used, reproduced in any manner whatsoever without written permission from the author, except in the case of brief quotations embodied in critical articles and reviews.

The Author of this book is solely responsible and liable for its content including but not limited to the views, representations, descriptions, statements, information, opinions and references ["Content"]. The Content of this book shall not constitute or be construed or deemed to reflect the opinion or expression of the Publisher or Editor. Neither the Publisher nor Editor endorse or approve the Content of this book or guarantee the reliability, accuracy or completeness of the Content published herein and do not make any representations or warranties of any kind, express or implied, including but not limited to the implied warranties of merchantability, fitness for a particular purpose. The Publisher and Editor shall not be liable whatsoever for any errors, omissions, whether such errors or omissions result from negligence, accident, or any other cause or claims for loss or damages of any kind, including without limitation, indirect or consequential loss or damage arising out of use, inability to use, or about the reliability, accuracy or sufficiency of the information contained in this book.

This Book is Dedicated to

my beloved late father-a true simple soul with a big heart,
my mother- for all her kindness and love- like an unchanged melody,
my younger brother Sudhir – for his honesty and righteousness,
my elder brother and his family,
my in-laws – for their kindness,
my lovely daughter Kartika and wife Jharna – for always
encouraging me and for being my strength,
Professor Rajesh Tiwari and all my friends

AND

To my teacher and mentor,
Professor Dinesh Kumar Pal,
for all the support, guidance and encouragement.

Contents

Foreword ix

Preface xi

Acknowledgements xiii

1. Brief Introduction to Epidemiology 1

    Defining Epidemiology 2

    Distribution and Determinants of Disease 4

    Key Characteristics of Epidemiology.......................7

    Uses of Epidemiology 8

    Component-Based Categories of Epidemiology 9

2. Public Health & Some Common Applications of Epidemiology ...11

    Epidemiology and Its Linkage with Public Health 12

    Understanding Causation of Disease 13

    Understanding the Natural History of Disease 14

    Describing Health Status of Populations..................15

    Evaluating Interventions 15

3. Disease and Some Key Concepts 21

    Levels of Existence of Disease 22

    Epidemic 23

    Epidemic Patterns 25

    Endemic 27

    Some Other Terms 28

4. Measurements Relating to Health & Disease 31
   Measurement of Morbidity 32
   Measurement of Mortality 39
   Burden of Disease-Some Concepts 51

5. Basic Approaches and Methods in Epidemiology 59
   The Work Epidemiologists Do 60
   Brief Introduction to Epidemiological Methods 61

6. Descriptive Epidemiology 65
   Steps Involved in Descriptive Studies 66
   Time, Person and Place Details and Their Use 78

7. Analytical Epidemiology 91
   Case-Control Studies 92
   Key Steps of Case-Control Studies 93
   Cohort Studies 104

8. Experimental Epidemiology 113
   Randomized Controlled Trials (RCTs) 115
   Non-Randomized Controlled Trials 123

9. Causation in Epidemiology 129
   Strength of Causal Factors 130
   Factors in Causation 131
   Establishing a Causal Relation 132
   Proving Causation 133

10. Screening for Disease 135
   Screening 137

11. Investigating an Epidemic 155
   Steps Involved in Investigating Epidemics 158

12. Public Health Surveillance 173

Key Characteristics of Surveillance................................175

Core Functions of a Surveillance System 178

Basic Types of Surveillance......................................180

Categorization of Surveillance Strategies Based on Specific Situations...182

References *185*

Index *197*

Foreword

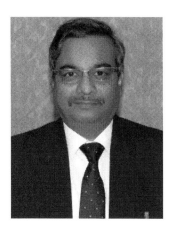

My association with Dr. Anil Mishra is very long, and I had the opportunity of being his guide and examiner for his post-graduation in Community Medicine. Since then he has been working in the field of public health and seen its ground level applications.

Over last few years I realized the intense desire that Dr. Anil Mishra had, for writing a book on epidemiology which simplistically narrates the concepts and makes it easier for the students at the undergraduate level to understand the basics of epidemiology.

In this book *'Basics of Epidemiology-Concepts made simple,'* Dr. Anil Mishra has successfully shaped his ideas into reality. The book is full of necessary examples and illustrations which give better clarity to understand key concepts. I am sure that this book will find a unique place in the minds of students, for developing conceptual clarity in basic epidemiology.

Foreword

I congratulate Dr. Anil Mishra for his untiring efforts for putting his ideas into reality through this book and wish him all the best in this endeavour.

With best wishes

Dr. Dinesh Kumar Pal
Professor & Head Department of Community Medicine,
Gandhi Medical College, Bhopal
And
Dean, Faculty of Medicine,
Madhya Pradesh Medical Science University, Jabalpur

Preface

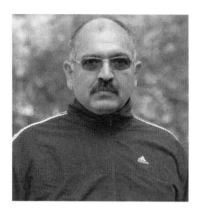

Epidemiology, which is a vital tool of the broader discipline of public health, needs a thorough conceptual clarity in the minds of medical graduates. This clarity will enable them to view health problems through a public health lens when they enter into the professional practice. Having a sound understanding of the fundamentals of epidemiology, in an application-based manner, is critical for strengthening public health systems and need-based rationalization of its approaches.

The current book 'Basics of Epidemiology-Concepts made Simple' has been developed keeping these very objectives and need of the time in mind. The books that are currently available and are usually referred to are voluminous and have the subject matter designed and presented to suit university question papers' pattern in mind.

Proper understanding of the basic concepts of epidemiology is paramount for medical graduates. Irrespective of the branch one selects for specialization, these basic concepts are required in research for even elementary analytics in medical science. Also, all medical professionals have to perform the role of public health physicians, with a specific focus on epidemiology, at some or other stage in their professional career. This book aims to provide clarity on concepts and basic methodological approaches in epidemiology from that perspective.

The content is mostly derived from guidelines of the World Health Organization (WHO) and Centre for Disease Control and Prevention (CDC). We are highly optimistic that the book will serve as a useful resource to help you develop clarity on the subject.

January, 2018 — Dr. Anil Mishra

Acknowledgements

It has been nearly two years I have been working on this book, and it is a satisfying feeling that the book is ready for the students. As happens with anyone, there were a lot of distractions when I either slowed down or even went off this task at times. My support system of family members, friends and my mentor and guide, helped me regain focus in such circumstances.

I feel blessed to have the valuable guidance of my mentor and teacher, Professor Dinesh Kumar Pal, on developing this book. In spite his hectic work schedule and administrative responsibilities, he always took out time for discussion and for reviewing individual chapters. I feel pleased to acknowledge the role Professor Rajesh Tiwari played in helping me move forward in the field of public health.

Different guidelines and publications from the Centre for Disease Control and Prevention (CDC), Atlanta and the World Health Organization (WHO) were of immense help in adding value to the subject matter. Similarly, referred publications from different authors and organizations were of great help in developing the subject material for individual chapters. I am personally indebted to them.

The book finally arrived into the present shape due to efforts from the Notion Press team, and I am thankful to them for giving it an impressive form.

I am also thankful to all the students who are going to use this book as their companion on basic epidemiology and will provide their valuable feedback for improving it further.

January 2018   Dr. Anil Mishra

CHAPTER 1

Brief Introduction to Epidemiology

Learning Objectives

- ❖ Develop conceptual clarity on what is epidemiology.
- ❖ Understand different terms used in the definition of epidemiology.
- ❖ Apprise yourself with the key characteristics of epidemiology.
- ❖ Understand the basics of distribution and determinants of disease.
- ❖ Know about the uses of epidemiology.
- ❖ Learn about functional categorization of key branches of epidemiology.

DEFINING EPIDEMIOLOGY

News reporters and journalists know that a good news story, whether it be about a crime, rescue or relief operations, or a public figure's statements or speech, should essentially be woven around the following 5 W's:

What,
Who,
Where,
When and
Why (why/how).

If the news is missing in any of these essential 5 W's, which are the basic components of a news story, the story is incomplete. The same approach is important when we describe health-related events, whether it be an outbreak of H1N1 influenza in India or spread of ZICA virus in any part of the world.

The connotations these 5Ws have about the study of diseases which afflict people, or other health outcomes, are closely related to 5 Ws stated above. Let's look at these related terms:

Diagnosis or health event (what),
Person (who),
Place (where),
Time (when), and
Causes, risk factors, and modes of transmission (why/how).[1]

The concept stated above is the foundation of the basic framework of the science of epidemiology. The term epidemiology is a derived from a combination of three words of Greek language:

Epi, meaning 'on' or 'upon',
Demos, meaning 'people' and
Logos, meaning the 'study of'[2]

In other words, the term epidemiology deals with the study of what befalls a population. Let us try to focus on this imaginary news shown on a Television Channel- *'An epidemic of Cholera has been reported from Dharavi, which is Asia's largest slum settlement in the city of Mumbai. Around 300 children and 60 adults have been affected. The first case was reported on 15 March, and many more cases were reported by 17th March. Investigations revealed that the water supply point from where the families of affected individuals were fetching drinking water was contaminated with sewage'.*

Try to check whether the reporter has captured all 'W's in this report. The statement above resembles an example of very basic epidemiological investigation finding.

Now, after some clarity about the basic concept, let us see the structured definition. There are many proposed, but looking at the underlying principles and the role epidemiology plays as a tool of public health, the following definition appears most relevant,

Epidemiology is the **study** *of the* **distribution** *and* **determinants** *of* **health-related states or events** *in* **specified populations** *and the* **application** *of this study to the control of health problems.*[1, 3]

Simplifying the Terms Used in the Definition:

For quick and complete understanding of the definition of epidemiology as given above, table 1 below explains the meaning of key terms used-[2]

Table 1: Key Terms Used in the Definition of Epidemiology

Meaning of Key Terms Used in the Definition of Epidemiology	
STUDY	It means any investigation of disease outbreak, surveillance, planned observations on health events, testing a proposed hypothesis, analytical research experiments
DISTRIBUTION	Any analysis to understand how a particular disease or health event is distributed, specifically regarding the timing of occurrence, persons, places affected.
DETERMINANTS	Important factors that are affecting the disease. These can be physical, chemical, biological, social, cultural, economic or behavioral factors.

Contd...

Meaning of Key Terms Used in the Definition of Epidemiology	
HEALTH-RELATED STATES/EVENTS	It means any disease or condition, behavior and related events, preventive, control or treatment interventions
SPECIFIED POPULATIONS	Meaning those who have specific characteristics, or are affected with or at risk of developing a disease, A few examples are adolescent girls, specific tribes, specific occupational groups, people with specific exposures (e.g., smokers), etc
APPLICATION FOR PREVENTION & CONTROL	Situation specific prevention, control or other remedial actions

DISTRIBUTION AND DETERMINANTS OF DISEASE

As the definition suggests, distribution and determinants of health-related events or states are the key focus area. Let us try to understand these in following sections.

Distribution

Distribution of diseases or health events can be over time, place or person. There are two key terms, i.e., Frequency and Pattern that are of importance here, let's understand them:

Frequency

It indicates how many numbers of times a particular health event, such as the number of cases of meningitis, diabetes, heat stroke or injectable drug abuse or any health-related event/outcome, was observed in a given population. It also reflects the relationship of that number to the size of the population. The resulting rate allows epidemiologists to compare disease occurrence across different populations. (e.g., prevalence of malnutrition in rural areas of India in comparison to urban areas)[1]

Pattern

Refers to the occurrence of health-related events by time, place, and person.

Time Patterns may be annual, seasonal, weekly, daily, hourly, weekday versus weekend or any other breakdown of time that may influence the occurrence of disease, health-related event or outcome. For example, malaria incidence in India peaks during monsoon months.[4]

Place Patterns include geographic variation, urban/rural differences, and location of work sites etc. For example, goitre used to be endemic in Himalayan and Tarai region of India, drunk driving peaks up during holidays.

Personal Characteristics include demographic factors, which may be related to the risk of illness, injury, disability or any other health related outcome or event, such as age, sex, marital status, and socioeconomic status, as well as behaviors and environmental exposures.[1] For example, it has been found that injectable drug users (IDUs) have a higher prevalence of HIV AIDS.

Characterizing health events by time, place, and person are activities of **descriptive epidemiology**, discussed in more detail later in this chapter.

Determinants

Determinants are defined as the underlying social, economic, cultural and environmental, genetic or other factors that play some role which is directly or indirectly responsible for health and disease. It is important to note that many of such factors do not belong to the field of health, rather they can be from sectors which influence health, for example, literacy.[5] These can be any single or group of factors, events, characteristic, or any definable entity, that brings about a change in a health condition. Determinants may also influence any other specified characteristic which in turn can bring changes in a health condition.[1]

Different categories of determinants have an important bearing on the health of the people. For example, children from poor socio-economic background have a high prevalence of undernutrition. Here, poor socio-economic status becomes one of the determinants.

Social determinants of health and their significance in tackling the disease burden have strongly been emphasized. The World Health Organization has set up a Commission on Social Determinants of Health which recommends to all nations for prioritizing actions to reduce health inequities arising because of social factors.[6] Epidemiologists have highlighted the role of these determinants in a large number of diseases and health outcomes.

'Epidemiologists assume that an illness does not occur randomly in a population, but happens only when the right accumulation of risk factors or determinants exists in an individual.'[1] Epidemiologists use **analytic epidemiology** or epidemiologic studies to discover and understand such factors (determinants), and to provide an explanation to questions like "Why this disease or health event is occurring" and "How is it caused?" They also try to assess if the population groups with different demographic or socio-cultural or economic characteristics, genetic or immunologic make-up, behaviors, environmental exposures or other potential factors show different rates of disease or health outcome. Ideally, the findings provide sufficient evidence to direct timely and effective public health control and prevention measures.[1]

In the points mentioned below, we have taken some examples that show the role of different determinants in the causation of disease or health events. Please read following sentences carefully and analyze:

1. Prolonged exposure to UV rays in the sunlight increases the risk of skin cancers. The risk is more to white-skinned people.
2. Muscular dystrophies have been found to have a genetic causation.
3. Trisomy of chromosome 21 is responsible for Down Syndrome.
4. The condition Haemophilia is typically caused by a hereditary lack of a coagulation factor, most often factor VIII.
5. Consumption of non-iodized salt is the main reason of Iodine Deficiency Disorders.
6. Carcinogens in the cigarette smoke are responsible for causing cancer of the lungs in chronic smokers.

All the above statements say something about 'How' and 'Why' of given diseases or medical conditions. Epidemiological studies help us arrive at such conclusions. We can very well understand how important these findings are if we want to check occurrence of a disease or medical conditions through various measures. Let's look at some important characteristics of epidemiology to understand this discipline and its scope in a broader context in the section below.

KEY CHARACTERISTICS OF EPIDEMIOLOGY

- It is a scientific discipline that makes use of sound methods of scientific inquiry into health-related events.
- It is a highly valuable scientific tool for public health which is data-driven. It relies on a systematic and unbiased approach to the collection, analysis, and interpretation of data, knowledge of probability, statistics, and sound research methods to arrive at conclusions.
- Basic epidemiologic methods rely on careful observation and comparative assessments. Such observations and assessments are carried out using valid comparison groups. The objective is to assess whether what was observed, such as the number of cases of a disease in a particular area during a particular time-period or the frequency of exposure to some specific factor among persons with disease, differs from what might be expected.[1]
- Epidemiology also draws on methods from other scientific fields, including biostatistics and informatics, biologic, economic, social, and behavioral sciences.
- It is a method of causal reasoning (what causes something) based on developing and testing scientifically grounded hypotheses to explain health-related behaviors, states, and events.
- Epidemiology is not merely a research activity but an integral component of public health, providing the foundation for directing practical and appropriate public health action through evidence-based science and causal reasoning.[1]

USES OF EPIDEMIOLOGY

The scientific descipline of epidemiology, and the information which various methods of epidemiology generate is of high importance in healthcare. There are numerous ways in which such information is used in healthcare and public health. Some of the common areas where epidemiology is used are:

- In the historical study of the health of a community and the rise and fall of diseases in the population and also for making disease trend projections into the future.
- For community diagnosis of the presence, nature, and distribution of health, events related to health, and diseases among the population. Subsequently, it is used to understand the dimensions of these events or diseases in terms of incidence, prevalence, and mortality, taking into consideration the dynamic nature any society has and also the dynamic nature that these health problems have.
- To study the working of health services beginning with the determination of needs and resources, proceeding to an analysis of services that are offered to meet such needs. Such studies are useful in making a comparison of the health status of different populations or their groups.
- To estimate the individual's chances and risk of getting diseases.
- To help complete the clinical picture by including all types of cases in proportion, by relating clinical disease to sub-clinical, by observing secular changes in the character of a disease, and its picture in other countries.
- In identifying syndromes from the distribution of clinical phenomena among sections of the population.
- In the search for causes of health and disease, starting with the discovery of groups with high and low rates, studying these differences in ways of living, and where possible, testing these notions to the actual practice among populations.[7]

COMPONENT-BASED CATEGORIES OF EPIDEMIOLOGY

In subsequent chapters, we will get into details of all these branches of epidemiology. At this stage, these are mentioned here just to introduce you to the concept.

Table 2: Some Key Categories of Epidemiology

Components	Category
Distribution • Distribution of disease over time • Distribution of disease over persons and places	DESCRIPTIVE EPIDEMIOLOGY
Determinants • Search for causes • Search for risk factors • Evaluate association of causal factors with disease/outcome (using different epidemiological methods)	ANALYTICAL EPIDEMIOLOGY
Individual Disease Outcome related epidemiological studies	DISEASE SPECIFIC EPIDEMIOLOGY
Applications (applying knowledge and practice of epidemiology to address public health issues)	APPLIED EPIDEMIOLOGY
Testing Hypothesis Proposed by epidemiological studies through experiments where the investigator can control and compare the outcome of exposure (e.g., clinical trials)	EXPERIMENTAL EPIDEMIOLOGY

Points to Remember

✤ Definition of epidemiology and its complete understanding.

✤ Understanding of all the key terms used in the definition of epidemiology.

✤ Key characteristics of the scientific discipline of epidemiology.

✤ Basic understanding on what ways the discipline of epidemiology is used.

✤ What are some key categories of epidemiology.

CHAPTER

2

PUBLIC HEALTH & SOME COMMON APPLICATIONS OF EPIDEMIOLOGY

Learning Objectives

- ❖ Acquire basic understanding on linkages of epidemiology with public health.
- ❖ Know how the descipline of epidemiology helps us in understanding causation of diseases.
- ❖ Get the basic idea on how epidemiology helps us determine a population's health status.
- ❖ Understand epidemiology's basic role in evaluating healthcare interventions.
- ❖ Get some idea about a few specialized branches of epidemiology.

EPIDEMIOLOGY AND ITS LINKAGE WITH PUBLIC HEALTH

Public health refers to the integrated actions (or collective actions) to improve the health of the population.[8] Epidemiology, which is one of the tools for improving public health, is used in several ways. Public health approaches are evidence-driven, and epidemiology finds that evidence. Early studies in epidemiology were concerned with the causes (aetiology) of communicable diseases, and such work continues to be essential since it can lead to the identification of methods of prevention for communicable diseases.[5] However, the role epidemiology plays in strengthening public health has tremendously evolved over time and now it plays a much bigger role.

Public health planning requires an understanding of the magnitude of different diseases. Not only this, but the patterns of disease distribution over persons, places and time are also needed to channelize efforts and resources in a rationalised and focused manner. Epidemiology also informs public health action in terms of evaluation of the risk factors, finding out which preventive or treatment approach is the best. With advances in technology and widening of knowledge base, newer treatments for different diseases keep developing. To evaluate such newer drugs, treatment methodologies or interventions, by comparing against the existing ones is a highly important work which is done through research using epidemiological methods.

When a new disease emerges, no one is aware of the natural history of such emerging diseases. It is the epidemiological research that tells us how is that disease caused, what is the agent, who are susceptible individuals, how is it transmitted, what are the risk factors, is there any genetic or molecular factor involved, so on and so forth.

In summary, we can conclude that whatever we do in public health or even in curative medicine, has its roots attached to epidemiology. Advancements in health care depend on this valuable tool of public health. Some of the broad functions, where there is direct and critically important application of epidemiology, are further detailed out as below-

UNDERSTANDING CAUSATION OF DISEASE

As we know, diseases have multifactorial causation. The interaction between the agent, host, and environment is critical. However, as per our understanding, some diseases are caused by genetic factors, examples include Haemophilia, Down's syndrome etc. There are many others for which an interaction between genetic and environmental factors is essential. Diabetes, for example, has both genetic and environmental components. Principally we know that the interactions of the agent, host and environment result in disease causation. We define environment broadly to include any biological, chemical, physical, psychological, economic or cultural factor that can affect health. Personal behaviours, also included in the host's environment, can further impact this interplay. Epidemiology is used to study the influence of such factors and also to analyse what is the best approach to prevent, control and treat such diseases.[5]

Almost every one of us would have heard or read the information 'cigarette smoking causes lung cancer.'[9] This is not known to us for eternity. Some researchers must have done a thorough analysis before this fact got established. In this statement, we see that there is a host, then there is a behaviour (smoking) and there are carcinogens in the cigarette smoke, i.e., the agent. The interplay among all these factors is resulting in lung cancer. The statement does not mean that a person who smoked one cigarette in life-time will have cancer of lungs. But, certainly there is an association and increasing risk with longer periods of smoking and so also with more number of cigarettes smoked per day. It is epidemiology which helps us arrive at such important facts through a variety of scientific methods.

The illustration below represents genetic factors, environmental factors and individual behaviours and the interplay of which has a multitude of effects on individuals' health. Such an interplay responsible for shifting the situation towards ill health from the state of good health. Epidemiologists work to find out which all factors are at play and are responsible for causation of a given disease.

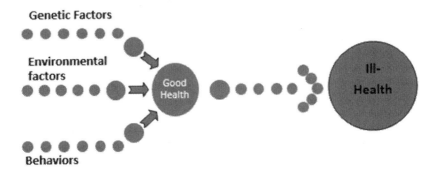

Figure 1: Schematic Representation of Factors Affecting Health

UNDERSTANDING THE NATURAL HISTORY OF DISEASE

In the illustration above (figure 1) we have seen that interplay of different factors affects an individual's health and it shifts towards ill health. For epidemiologists, details of this shift also matter. It is of interest to them to examine how a disease develops and progresses, what are the subclinical changes that occur in the host's body, how a disease clinically presents, what are the chances of a patient dying from a disease and what causes that ill person to die. Also matters the information like how many of patients are at the risk of dying from a disease and how many will recover. In those who recover what are the residual impairments, if there are any, and what proportion of individuals is likely to get such residual impairments.[5]

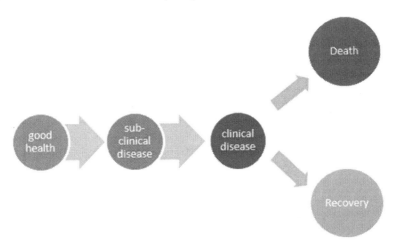

Figure 2: Shift from Good Health to ill Health

All this information related to the shift from good health to illness, as mentioned above and depicted in figure 2, is immensely useful. This forms the basis for developing public health strategies to prevent the occurrence of disease, reduce the harm caused if the disease occurs. Also, such knowledge is used to develop control strategies so that the spread of disease is minimized, and to develop most effective treatments, save affected people from dying and minimize and manage residual impairments left in the survivors. Majority of this work comes under the field of clinical epidemiology, which applies research on the natural history of disease for improving the physicians' diagnostic accuracy and ability to effectively treat patients in their regular clinical practice.[10]

DESCRIBING HEALTH STATUS OF POPULATIONS

Any government or its health system would want to have a regular update on the state of health of its people. Understanding the burden of diseases is important for planning and developing strategies to reduce that burden, and allocating required resources. Also, in some settings, there are specific exposures to chemical, physical, biological factors that predispose the local population to the risk of developing specific diseases. In such settings specific epidemiological studies, to evaluate and describe the problems in details, are of paramount importance. These studies and their findings help authorities take specific actions to safeguard people's health against the harmful effects of those exposures.[5]

If such assessments of population's health status are done periodically, then we can know about the trends over time and thus can make adjustments in our strategies accordingly. It will also be helpful to make changes in prevention and control strategies in case of diseases that show seasonal or other types of short-term fluctuations.

EVALUATING INTERVENTIONS

The World Health Organization in one of its evaluation report stated that 'the success of the OPV (Oral Polio Vaccine) in curtailing polio epidemics and reducing, or even eliminating the disease in endemic countries provides overwhelming evidence of the effectiveness of polio vaccines, in particular, OPV.[11] In drawing such inferences, epidemiology plays a highly important role.

We now have an understanding of the average duration of different diseases and the probable period of hospitalization needed. Clinicians will also be able to tell their patients about the efficacy of new drugs. Oncologists tell their patients about the survival rate for the cancer someone has and the effect different treatment regimen have on survival rates.

Let's see a valuable piece of information on diarrhoeal disease in India, gathered through highly valuable epidemiological studies, mentioned below, and try to see how epidemiology helps us in evaluating interventions:

> *'India has made steady progress in reducing deaths in children younger than five years, with total deaths declining from 2.5 million in 2001 to 1.5 million in 2012'.[12] This remarkable reduction was possible due to the inception and success of many universal programs like the expanded program on immunization, program for the control of diarrheal diseases and acute respiratory infection. Even though the deaths among children under-5 years have declined, the proportional mortality accounted by diarrheal diseases remains high. Diarrhoea is the third most common cause of death in under-five children, responsible for 13% deaths in this age-group, killing an estimated 300,000 children in India each year.[13] Information on diarrheal diseases, its determinants in India and preventive and control strategies in light of recent developments need to be reviewed for better planning and organization of health services within the community'.[13, 14]*

Similarly, information on facts like what percentage of lives of neonates and infants can be saved through early initiation and exclusive breastfeeding for six months, how institutional deliveries affect maternal mortality, what impact access to safe drinking water will have on childhood diarrhoea, to what extent full immunization coverage of children can bring down under five mortality etc. are all results of epidemiological investigations. Also, it helps us gain knowledge on areas like like the value of treating high blood pressure, the efficiency of sanitation measures to control diarrhoeal diseases etc.[15] Such information is valuable and is helpful in ensuring that a person having ill health is restored to the state of good health and also in cutting down numbers of preventable deaths.

The following illustration (figure 3) shows that whenever there is an illness in a community, the health system works on some principles. These are:

1. Establish correct diagnosis and start appropriate treatment
2. Advice people on general health promotion
3. Protect other susceptible people in the community from getting the disease through specific prevention and control measures.

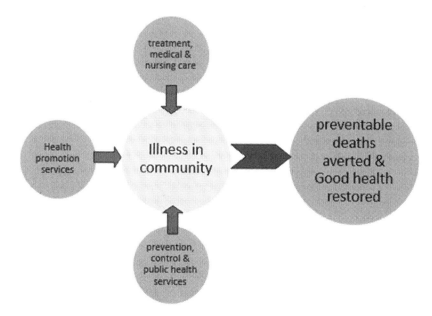

Figure 3: Actions Approach During Illnesses

To accomplish the tasks as represented in the illustration (figure 3) above, we will need information on the clinical and epidemiological features of the disease and also about the most effective treatment option. We need to know who are the susceptible hosts so that we can protect them using specific measures. The information on how a particular disease spreads/occurs will help us stop its transmission/occurrence.

While discussing some common applications of epidemiology in public health, in the paragraphs above, we realize that there are some specific fields. Treatment and outcome related studies come under **clinical epidemiology** disciplines. Some examples would be; studying appropriate length of stay in the hospital for specific conditions, the value of treating high blood pressure, the efficiency of sanitation measures to control diarrhoeal diseases etc.[15] There are other areas like genetic factors' involvement in disease causation which will come under **genetic epidemiology**. Genetic epidemiology involves studies to understand aetiology, distribution, manifestations, prevention and control of diseases that run in the families or relatives, including the disorders that are inheritable.[16] This field also tries to understand the responsible gene, the alterations, aberrations or mutations in specific locations that are responsible for disease causation. Upon exposure to external agents (chemicals, pathogenic organisms etc.) host's body response occurs through some molecular mechanisms. Concepts of epidemiology when applied to this area, fall into the category of **molecular epidemiology**. It involves evaluating host characteristics mediating the response to the external agents and also using biochemical markers to analyse specific effects of the disease process.[17] As we know that any drug that comes for use on population, undergoes rigorous experiments to study the desired therapeutic effects, side effects etc. Some drugs, which are in use, are also evaluated and recommendation about their use are made to the clinicians. All these come under the field of **pharmacoepidemiology**. Pharmacoepidemiology concentrates on clinical patient outcomes from therapeutics by using methods of clinical epidemiology and applying them to understanding the determinants of beneficial and adverse drug effects, the impact of genetic variation on drug effect, duration-response relationships, clinical effects of drug-drug interactions, and the effects of medication non-adherence.[18] Refer table 3 to see these details in brief;

Table 3: Activities Under Molecular and Genetic Epidemiology

Field	Activities
Molecular Epidemiology	Measuring exposure to specific substances and early biological response by 1. Evaluating host factors that mediate such response to external agents 2. Making use of specific biochemical markers to understand such changes
Genetic Epidemiology	Study diseases that occur in families, relatives to understand 1. Etiology 2. Distribution 3. Common manifestations Research in the field is aimed to identify and establish the responsible genetic factor and to understand the defects/alterations that cause the disease.

 Points to Remember

- How are public health and epidemiology are linked with one another? (Conceptual clarity).

- Role epidemiology plays in understanding causation of diseases (Conceptual clarity).

- How is natural history of a disease is deciphered with the help of epidemiology (Conceptual clarity).

- In what way epidemiology helps us in evaluating public health interventions (Conceptual clarity).

CHAPTER
3

DISEASE AND SOME KEY CONCEPTS

Learning Objectives

- ❖ Understanding about levels of existence of a disease.
- ❖ Know about the concept of 'Epidemics'.
- ❖ Learn about different patterns of epidemics.
- ❖ Understand what is an endemic.

In your public health lessons, you must have understood the basic concept of what is disease and how it is caused. If not, then refer to your public health textbook and try to understand that concept fully.

In this chapter, we will try to understand some more concepts about disease existence and its levels, and also about its transmission.

LEVELS OF EXISTENCE OF DISEASE

Every health system will try and make all possible efforts to eliminate diseases. Plenty of resources are put into the measures directed towards this objective. Such efforts are essential as diseases become public health problems and have a strong negative impact on the productivity of the individuals, families, societies, provinces or states, and nations at large.

It would be impractical to say that public health efforts focus on eliminating every single disease that affects us. Physicians try to treat individual diseases so that the person affected is able to restore her or his normal health and productivity. Public health at the population level, focuses on routine health promotional, prevention, and treatment strategies so that disease burden is reduced. For prioritizing action targeted to control a particular disease, understanding its level of existence is important. Equally important is to understand its distribution over places, persons and time. This is done through descriptive epidemiological studies.[1]

Public health system faces the challenge if -

- ➢ There is an occurrence of even a single case of a new disease or of a disease that had been eliminated,
- ➢ Cases of a disease exceed the expected numbers that occur routinely,
- ➢ Some disease persistently exists at a higher level in a geographic location,

As we know, for many diseases that are mild, there is a level to which they exist but do not pose a major problem to public health systems.

In the above context, let us now look at some specific terms that indicate the disease existence scenario in a community;

EPIDEMIC

We have discussed in preceding paragraphs that many diseases routinely exist to a certain level. In an ideal scenario, there should be no disease, but the practical observations indicate that there is a routine level of certain diseases occurring in any given population. If this level is minimal and does not pose a threat to the public health, then we take it as the parameter for comparison or the baseline, or routinely existing levels. Undoubtedly, efforts need to continue to reduce this routine occurrence also to a minimum achievable or zero level, as we have achieved, for example, in case of smallpox. The diseases like chickenpox, measles and many more, continue to occur to a certain level in different populations.

Whenever the level occurrence of any disease exceeds the routinely expected level, we call it an epidemic. It can happen because of a variety of factors. Some key situations when this occurs are-

- If any disease-causing organism's ability to cause disease increases or its presence increases.
- If environmental factors favour rapid multiplication of the organism and its spread or they increase presence or concentration of other disease-causing agents in the hosts' environment.
- When the size of susceptible population pool increases or the population's exposure to a particular risk factor increases.

In case of non-communicable diseases also, the term epidemic is equally applicable. When the size of the population pool that is exposed to a particular risk factor increases, or the health promotional and preventive strategies don't work, it results into increased chances of an epidemic of a non-communicable disease happening. For example, more people start smoking cigarettes, or those who are already smokers increase the number of cigarettes they smoke every day, more people start living stressful lives or the level of stress increases etc. Such situations are likely to result in epidemics of non-communicable diseases like hypertension and other cardiovascular diseases, mental disorders, lung cancer etc.[5]

While using the term epidemic, we need to remember that it often implies, specifically in relation to infectious diseases, a rapid increase of the number of cases of a disease or an event in a defined population. So, the time and geographical (place) factors are always considered.

Commonly, we find terms like **outbreak** used in epidemiological investigations and reports. This term also carries the same meaning as the term *epidemic* does, but it's particularly used in context to a smaller geographic area, for example, an *outbreak of measles in a village*.[1]

Now, after having understood the meaning of the term epidemic, next fundamental point is to understand, to what degree the increase in the numbers of cases of a disease must be there to be labelled as an epidemic. This is a judgement that health authorities have to make. As we discussed earlier, this judgment depends upon multiple factors and varies from disease to disease. For a disease that has been eliminated from a geographical location, the occurrence of even a single case needs utmost attention, and this needs to be treated as an epidemic. For diseases that are either very serious, have a low incidence and prevalence, a small increase in cases over the baseline level should be labelled as an epidemic. Sometimes, health authorities have to respond to even a small number of cases, depending upon the seriousness of the diseases, the vulnerability of the population involved and considering the degree of public health threat that disease poses.

It is important to remember that the prime importance is to investigate the occurrence of all cases which can pose a serious threat to public health, irrespective whether we could label it as an epidemic or not. This investigation further gives us many clues. Many times, we notice an increase in the number of cases of a disease when reporting network improves. Contrary to this we can see a reduction in the numbers of cases if a fairly large segment of the population migrates out of a particular geography. Erroneous reporting, misdiagnosis, migration, lack of correct data for comparison are some reasons that can present a confusing situation. Therefore, public health should always rely on the proper epidemiological investigations to arrive at any conclusion about this. Certainly, there are situations where an increase in the number of cases reported creates no ambiguity, and we can label this as an epidemic.

EPIDEMIC PATTERNS

Based on the origin and different course patterns of epidemics, we can categorize them into following groups:[1]

- Common source epidemic
- Propagated epidemics
- Mixed epidemics
- Others

Common Source Epidemics or Outbreaks

As the name suggests, there is a common source from which all people affected got the disease. Now, there can be two scenarios in common source outbreaks. One, where all affected individuals were exposed for a very brief period and after that the source was no longer passing on the disease (the term 'infection' is more appropriate and relevant in this example). For example, in a dinner party, the ice-cream served was contaminated with Salmonella. All people who ate this fell ill within one incubation period. This is an example of a *common point source outbreak.*[1]

Let us look at a little different scenario. Suppose a drinking water supply tank is contaminated with E. coli and those getting water to drink from it are falling ill due to E. coli diarrhoea. The contaminated water is being supplied to a community on a continuous basis. Since the source is common and nature of passing on the infection causing organism is continuous, hence the name *common continuous source outbreak.*

There can be one more type of common source outbreak, and that is *intermittent common source outbreak.* This occurs when the exposure to the disease-causing agent is intermittent in nature. Increased number of cases coincide with the incubation period following the periods of high exposure, and these numbers fall following low exposure periods (or when there is no exposure).[1]

Propagated Epidemics

These types of epidemics occur in a situation where the disease propagates from person to person.[1] Most commonly, these are caused due to direct person to person spread (example, measles), but there can be vehicles (like shared syringes which spread HIV or Hepatitis B among injectable drugs users- from one infected individual to others). Whenever a new person is infected, manifestations of the disease develop following the incubation period. So, the spread to multiple individuals happens involving multiple incubation periods.

In propagated epidemics, when a case spreads the disease to a smaller group of his or her close contacts, the number of cases are usually not very large. But, when the primary contacts of the original index case get infected and then all of them, in turn, start infecting their contacts and the number now begin to grow in somewhat exponential manner, as illustrated in figure 4 below;

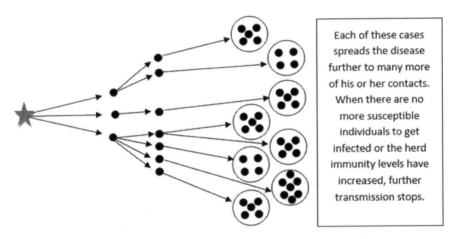

Figure 4: Illustration showing exponential increase in cases in propagated epidemics

In propagated epidemics, there is an increase in the number of cases following multiple incubation periods. But, after a stage, when there are no more susceptible contacts who can get infected, it reaches a plateau. This can happen either because the herd immunity is developed, or proper prevention and control measures are instituted. The number, after this stage, will come down if the infected individuals are properly treated, and they no longer remain active to pass on the disease to others.[1, 5]

Mixed Epidemics

In this type of epidemics, we can see that some individuals get the disease from a common source, and then they start spreading it to their contacts through person to person transmission.[1]

Other Types

If we see the examples of vector-borne diseases or zoonotic diseases then we realize that these fit neither into the common source and nor into propagated types of epidemics. There should be favourable conditions for the spread of diseases in terms of a sufficient number of cases among hosts. Also, there should be a sufficient number of vectors involved and also the environment where the host and vector interactions happen frequently, i.e., these vectors come in contact with human hosts. This means that there has to be a human-animal-environment interface or human-vector-environment interface for such diseases to spread. For example, cases of malaria in a community will not be able to transmit the disease to other people through person to person contact. There has to be the presence of mosquitoes in the environment and also their interaction with other individuals (biting) for the disease to spread. Similarly, for rabies to spread to humans, rabid carnivores or bats should have interactions with them (bites, licks).[1]

ENDEMIC

The term endemic means there is a constant presence of an event or health condition or a disease in a geography. Under ideal conditions, health systems anywhere would not want diseases to exist persistently in a geography. But, many events, health conditions or diseases persist at somewhat constant level because of a variety of reasons. Often, these levels are considered as the baseline for evaluating if there is further increase or decrease. The levels of occurrence of these events, health conditions or diseases are comparatively high in terms of incidence and prevalence in endemic areas in comparison non-endemic areas (for that particular event, health condition or disease).[1]

There are situations where public health authorities, on assumptions that the disease occurrence is not going to affect all susceptible individuals in the community, may not carryout any interventions. In such conditions, the disease would continue to occur, at the same level, indefinitely. If the conditions become more favourable then the number of cases will start increasing. Interactions between the agent, host and environment go on resulting in occurrence of disease. Through interventions, we make attempts to change the dynamics of these interactions and make conditions less favourable for the disease to spread.

SOME OTHER TERMS

In some geographies, a particular disease may exist persistently at very high levels. This situation of endemicity of a disease is known as **Hyperendemic**.[3] Whether the levels of a disease are high or low will be decided in the context of usual occurrence of that disease in the given geography.

Holoendemic is another important term. It means a high level of infection starting at a young age (childhood) that involves the majority of susceptible individuals in that age group, the adult population also shows the evidence of disease but in lower proportions. Also, the obvious manifestations of the disease, or signs of damage caused by it, are much less in adult population because of adaptive immunity developed in them against that disease.[3, 19]

The term **pandemic** denotes a larger picture, meaning, the condition where a disease becomes endemic for large geographical areas like the entire continent or regions involving many countries.[20]

You must have heard the term **sporadic** while reading public health. This refers to a disease that occurs infrequently and irregularly, or is scattered over places and time. A sporadic disease may change into an epidemic or endemic depending upon the local conditions that support its spread, or those favouring its persistence in the area. For a disease that has been uprooted, or some new diseases not noticed before in a given area, even a sporadic occurrence is alarming. Under any of these situations, a thorough epidemiological investigation is needed.[1]

 Points to Remember

- Concept of levels of existence of disease.
- Epidemic-the concept.
- Common source epidemics.
- Propagated epidemics.
- Mixed epidemics.
- Endemic-the concept.
- Hyperendemic- the concept.
- Holoendemic-the concept.
- Pandemic-the concept.
- Sporadic disease-the concept.

CHAPTER 4

Measurements Relating to Health & Disease

Learning Objectives

- Learn about principles and most commonly used indices for measuring morbidity.
- Undestand how is mortality measured and what are some key concepts related to indices for measuring mortality.
- Familiarise yourself with most commonly used mortality rates and ratios.
- Understand basics about the concept of 'burden of disease'.
- Learn about two important concepts related to disease burden, i.e. Disability Adjusted Life Years (DALYs) and Quality Adjusted Life Years (QALYs).

As we know, understanding the health situation of a population is one of the core functions of epidemiology. For this purpose, certain measurements would be essential. These measurements are related to general health, its deterioration towards illness and the outcomes of illness, i.e., recovery, disability or death. The underlying objective of these measurements is always to tailor the most appropriate interventions to control different diseases and restore the productivity of individuals.

When we try to measure something, then we would want clear information on what is to be measured, precisely. Let us now look at the standard WHO definition of Health- "health is a state of complete physical, mental, and social well-being and not merely the absence of disease or infirmity."[21]

Now, the challenge is how to measure well-being. There are so many variables to define it. Therefore, in practice, the epidemiologists will have to resort to simpler and practical definitions. Let us say, for practical purposes, an individual who has no disease (or systemic complaint) and has all normal bodily functions would be considered 'healthy' for such purpose. Such relaxations in the practical definitions are acceptable, as far as the health measurements are concerned. However, when it comes to measurement of morbidity or mortality, we have specific indices which are clearly defined. We will go through the key indices in subsequent paragraphs.

MEASUREMENT OF MORBIDITY

In simplest terms, morbidity means any deviation from health. It is synonymous with sickness, illness or disease.[22] Public health endeavors aim to bring back persons from the conditions of morbidity to good health. This is achieved through instituting appropriate measures of control and treatment. It is always essential to understand which population is at risk of developing a particular disease and what is the level of that risk. These indices of morbidity help us in making such assessments.

Population at Risk

The population at risk is the population that is exposed to the occurrence of a vital event.[23] It is worth noting here that while instituting the measures of prevention and control we must clearly understand which population sub-group is at the risk. For a condition that occurs in children only, if we try to cover adults and elderly too with those measures then certainly it is a waste of time, resources, and energy. It is a fault or misunderstanding in our planning. Similarly, for measures aimed towards cancer of ovaries, we cannot think of covering men with these measures. Therefore, the most basic step is to understand the susceptible population for a given disease condition.

In a nutshell, a given set or subset of a population that is susceptible to a certain disease becomes the 'population at risk' for that particular disease.

Indices of Measurement

We have some important indices that we use for measuring the diseases or health-related characteristics in a population. We will see those in the following sections, one by one.

Let us take the example of Tuberculosis. We all know that there are some existing old cases of this disease in a given population. Then there are some susceptible people who come in contact with existing active cases and get infected and develop tuberculosis. So, in this scenario, we have some pre-existing cases and some new cases.

We can take the example of non-communicable diseases also. Diabetes Mellitus has some pre-existing and some new cases. The same will hold true for attributes like smoking, there are some existing smokers in a community and seeing them some new people start smoking. By analyzing this information, you can say how many new smokers add up to a population during a given period and how many already exist. For having an idea of the total number of smokers who exist in a community on a given day (let us take it as 'today') – we must gather information on the number of people who smoke, which will include people who have been smoking since years as well as those who started smoking later or at any time till today. But, if we want to see how many new smokers started smoking this year then, we will have to discard the smokers who started smoking before beginning of this year.

Let us try to see two important terms, incidence and prevalence, in the above context. In the above example, **Incidence** means all new smokers who added up during a given period (say 'this year'). It will include only those who started smoking in the given period. Whereas, **prevalence,** in this example of smokers, would mean 'all smokers', old as well as new, who are smoking during that reference period or at that point.

As we know, the incidence and prevalence vary from disease to disease. There may be low incidence and high prevalence situations – as for diabetes – or a high incidence and low prevalence situation – as for the common cold. Colds occur more frequently than diabetes but last only a short time, whereas diabetes is a lifelong condition.

Incidence

The "incidence" of a condition is the number of new cases in a time period – usually one year.[24]

Calculating Incidence

Let us assume that we are discussing disease 'X'

Incidence takes into account the variable time periods during which individuals are disease-free and thus "at risk" of developing the disease.

The numerator (the top number in a fraction) is new events of disease 'X' during a given period.

Denominator (the bottom number in a fraction) is the population at risk (of having disease 'X') during the same period as above.

$$\text{Incidence} = \frac{\text{Number of new cases of disease occurring in a given period}}{\text{Population at risk during the same period}} \quad (5)$$

The units of incidence rate must always include a unit population size and that of time (cases per unit population size as appropriate and per week/month/year, etc. depending upon the period of observation).

For example, if you have observed a village of population 5000 for one week and found that there were 185 new cases of diarrhoea that occurred during that period of observation, then we can say 'incidence of diarrhoea is **37 cases per 1000 population per week (for that particular week)**

$$Incidence = \frac{185}{5000} \times 1000 = 37 \text{ cases per 1000 population during the given week}$$

Using appropriate units of the population is convenient for understanding. In the above example, we calculated the incidence for 1000 population. We can express it as a percentage by multiplying with 100 in place of 1000 in the above example.

Let us assume that a survey was conducted to find out new cases of some rare disease that occurred during a year and only one case was found in the surveyed population of 80,000. Under this situation, it would be appropriate and easy to understand, if we report this incidence per 100,000 population to get value which is above 1 at least.

$$Incidence = \frac{1}{80,000} \times 100000 = 1.25 \text{ per 100,000 population per year (given year).}$$

It helps us quickly make the judgment that we can get 5 cases of this rare disease for roughly 400,000 population every year.

Prevalence

Prevalence is the proportion of persons in a population who have a particular disease or attribute at a specified point in time or over a specified period.[1, 5] Prevalence differs from incidence in that prevalence includes all cases, both new and pre-existing, in the population at the specified time, whereas incidence is limited to new cases only.

When you collect this information in reference to a particular point of time, this is known as **Point Prevalence** and is defined as the proportion of a population that has the characteristic at a specific point in time.[1, 25]

This point does not necessarily mean the exact minute, hour or day. It may extend beyond that. For example, trying to see how many children are suffering from upper respiratory infections during a week in the peak of winters. Here the 'point' extends into a week. This will include those children also, who are having a respiratory infection that started even before the beginning of that week.

Another way is to measure the prevalence is **Period Prevalence,** which refers to prevalence measured over an interval of time. It is the proportion of persons with a particular disease or an attribute at any time during the specified interval.[1, 25] For example, if we want to know how many cases of hepatitis B are *existing and occurring* in the year 2016, then we will consider the period 01st January 2016 to 31st December 2016.

The numerator will always be 'the total number of cases of that particular disease (old and new)' but the reference to time frame would be different.

Calculating Prevalence

$$\text{Point Prevalence (of disease A)} = \frac{\text{Total cases of disease A (old plus new) at a given point in time}}{\text{Estimated population at risk of disease A at that point of time}} \times 100$$

$$\text{Period Prevalence (of disease B)} = \frac{\text{Total cases of disease B (old plus new) during given period.}}{\text{Estimated mid-period population at risk of disease B}} \times 100$$

The illustration (figure 5) below explains this further;

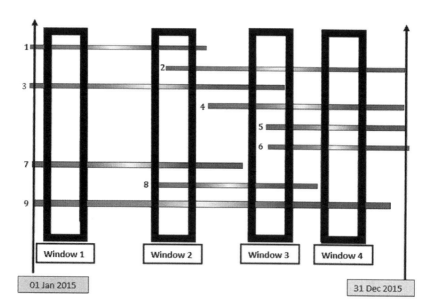

Figure 5: Illustration explaining incidence and prevalence

On seeing the illustration above (figure 5), we observe that there are cases which are pre-existing and at the same time there are cases which are new, beginning in the given period. In other words, we find cases in different stages. When we look at window 1 (point of time), then we notice that there are 4 cases which are pre-existing and no new cases reported during this point of time (which is represented by window 1). Window 2 shows 6 cases, four old and two new ones; window 3 shows 7 cases out of which two are detected to begin at that point of observation. Window 4 shows a total of 5 cases.

Now overlook the individual windows and try to see how many cases (old and new) were there between period 1st January 2015 and 31st December 2015. There are total nine cases.

So, what is the inference? We can see that in the point prevalence we run the risk of missing some cases, specifically in case of those diseases which do not have a very long duration. No doubt, the point prevalence gives us a quick snapshot of the situation at a given point in time. But, it does not give us a complete picture.

Relation Between Incidence and Prevalence

Let us now try to understand the relation between incidence and prevalence. To do that we will take a hypothetical example of a disease which has an average duration of three years. Now, imagine that the incidence of this disease was 20 cases per year for the given population. It means that all twenty new cases which occurred in any year will last for three years, assuming that all survive through this period.

Table 4: Explaining relationship between incidence and prevalence

	Yr. 2007	Yr. 2008	Yr 2009	Yr. 2010	Yr.2011	Yr. 2012	Yr.2013	Yr. 2014	Yr. 2015		
Yr. 2007	20 new cases in the year										
Yr. 2008		20 new cases in the year									
Yr 2009			20 new cases in the year								
Yr. 2010				20 new cases in the year							
Yr.2011					20 new cases in the year						
Yr. 2012						20 new cases in the year					
Yr.2013							20 new cases in the year				
Yr. 2014								20 new cases in the year			
Yr. 2015									20 new cases in the year		
Prevalence			60	60	60	60	60	60	60		
Incidence		Assumed to be 20 cases per year for the period 2007 to 2015									

If we carefully look at table 4 above, we understand that the cases originating in a year last for three years, as the duration of that disease is three years. Similarly, there are cases which originated earlier and lasted for three years. When we look any column between the year 2009 and 2015, then we find that for any individual year column, there are new cases[20] for that year and there are cases from preceding 2 years (40 cases) which increase the total number of cases (to 60).

Let's now see, what the relationship is between prevalence and incidence -

Prevalence = Incidence of disease X mean duration of disease[5]

In the above example, the incidence is 20 cases per year (for the years 2007 to 2015) and mean duration is three years, hence-

Prevalence = 20 X 3 = 60,

Now, examine individual columns for years 2009 to 2015 (enclosed inside the box with thick border). For every column, we see there are three highlighted cells, each of which represents 20 cases, i.e., the value of incidence, thus making the total 60 for new and pre-existing cases for that year, i.e., the prevalence.

MEASUREMENT OF MORTALITY

In almost every country there is a population-based system of registration of births and deaths. The problems associated with such systems are missed events, delayed registration and inability to register correct cause of death. In deaths which do not occur in institutions, it becomes difficult to ascertain the exact cause.

Even in specialized institutions having the qualified workforce, sometimes, there are situations when they fail to arrive at the exact cause. We may find a patient getting treated on wrong lines, as the diagnosis made was incorrect.

In any situation, to understand the impact or fatality of a disease, we will need to know how many of total deaths are caused by that particular disease. Epidemiologists do such estimations using certain indices which are discussed below;

Indices of Measurement

Crude Death Rate

Before we arrive at specific causes, we need to have a sense of the total number of deaths taking place in a defined geographical area. The means to do that is calculating a Crude Death Rate (CDR). This is defined as the number of deaths occurring in the population of a given geographical area during a given year, per 1,000 mid-year total population of the same geographical area during the same year.[26]

Let's understand the steps to estimate crude death rate. In a defined geography, we will need to know all deaths taking place in all age groups, all sexes, due to all causes, in a defined period, say one year. This becomes the numerator. Now, we need the number of people who are exposed to the risk of dying (denominator) to know the proportion. Every person in that population is assumed to be at the risk of dying. Hence we take into account the entire mid-year population.

In this example, the entire population living in that particular area becomes susceptible population. In the given year, the population of the given area is likely to undergo some changes. Population between 01st January and 31st December of that year is unlikely to remain the same. Therefore, we take mid-year population as it eliminates the bias which may arise if we take the population of one or the other extreme of the year.

$$\text{Crude Death Rate} = \frac{\text{Total number of deaths occurring during a year}}{\text{Estimated mid-year population in that year}} \times 10^n$$

We see the multiplication factor '10^n' written in the formula above. For example, an area having population 50,000 reported 300 deaths in a given year, let us try calculating the crude death rate for per thousand population (here, '10^n' -becomes 10^3 i.e. 1000);

$$\text{Crude Death Rate} = \frac{300}{50,000} \times 1000 = 6 \text{ per } 1000$$

It is always necessary to mention specifically whether the calculation is for per 100 or per 1000, per 10,000 or per 100,000 population.

Now, let us try to understand the concepts of some specific measures of mortality. We will begin with Cause-Specific Death Rate for discussion.

Cause-Specific Death Rate

This is a highly important indicator that gives us an understanding of the impact, in terms of mortality, caused by a given medical condition/cause. We know that for any population, there is a system of recording all deaths with specific mention of the cause.

If we take the example of road traffic accidents. From the causes for individual death records we can know how many deaths have resulted from road traffic accidents. Let us consider that a state of India (hypothetical example) that has an estimated mid-year (2014) population of 6 crores (60000000) and in that year, i.e. in 2014, there were total 4, 80,000 deaths for all ages and sexes combined. Out of these, 180,000 were due to road traffic accidents.

From the concept of cause-specific mortality rate we already know that it is the total number of deaths due to a given specific cause (road traffic accidents, in our example) in a given year for the mid-year population in that particular year.[1] We need to understand the numerator and denominator in the formula below clearly-

$$\text{Cause-specific mortality rate} = \frac{\text{Number of deaths in the given population due to a specific cause in a given year}}{\text{Estimated mid-year population for the given year}} \times 10^n$$

We will now put the values from our hypothetical example and try to calculate the rate

$$\text{Road traffic accident specific Mortality} = \frac{180000}{60000000} \times 1000 = 3 \text{ deaths}/1000 \text{ population}$$

We can express this rate for 1000 population, 10,000 or 100000 population if required.

Proportionate Mortality

We will now try to derive one more information from the example above, and that is about Proportionate Mortality. Proportionate mortality describes the proportion of deaths in a specified population over a period attributable to different causes.[1] So, from the above example, we know that out of 480000 total deaths in the year 2014, 180000 deaths occurred due to road traffic accidents. This also means that 480000-180000= 300000 deaths occurred due to causes other than road accidents. Using simple calculation, we can find out the proportion of deaths due to road traffic accidents:

$$\text{Proportionate mortality of road accidents} = \frac{180000}{480000} \times 100 = 37.5\%$$

Here is the technically correct wording of the formula for calculating proportionate mortality (for a given cause, for a given population, for a given period)-

$$= \frac{\text{Death due to the specific cause in a given population in the given period}}{\text{All deaths due to all cases in the same population \& same period}} \times 100$$

Proportionate mortality is always expressed as a percentage, and if we add up the proportions of all deaths in a given population over a given period due to different causes, it should sum up to 100%, provided no information about the cause of death is missing.

Death to Case Ratio

There is also a need to understand how lethal different diseases are. To do that we follow a concept of Death to Case Ratio, which is defined as the number of deaths attributed to a particular disease during a specified period divided by the number of new cases of that disease identified during the same period.[1]

From the public health point of view, as well as for a clinician, it is highly important to understand which disease has higher chances of taking lives of those who get affected by such a disease. It guides us to pay high emphasis on taking adequate preventive measures in time and also gives clinicians an indication to take appropriate curative measure promptly with needed aggressiveness. It is a common sense based derivation. Let us understand it with a simple imaginary example- In the year 2015, country 'A' reported 1000 new cases of disease X and in the same year there were deaths of 200 patients suffering from the disease X. The same country in the same year had 500 new cases of disease Y and death of 150 patients who had this disease Y. Now, first of all, we will look at the formula for calculating **Death to Case Ratio.**

$$\text{Death to Case Ratio (Disease X)} = \frac{\text{Number of deaths assigned to disease X in a given period}}{\text{Number of new cases of disease X that occurred in the same period}}$$

Putting values in the formula for disease X from our example above, will further simplify it;

$$\text{Death to Case Ratio (Disease X)} = \frac{200 \text{ (deaths due to disease X in the year 2015)}}{1000 \text{ (new cases of disease X reported in 2015)}}$$

$$\text{Death to Case Ratio (Disease X)} = \frac{200}{1000} = 2/10 \text{ i.e. 2 deaths for every 10 new cases}$$

OR

$$\text{Death to Case Ratio (Disease X)} = \frac{200}{1000} \times 100 = 20 \text{ deaths for every 100 new cases}$$

Undoubtedly, these 200 deaths occurred in the year 2015. However, some of these 200 deaths must have been in the cases which had onset in the preceding years and not in 2015. But the denominator (all new cases in 2015) is confined to 2015. Hence, we can NOT say that in the year 2015, 20 patients out of 100 new reported cases of disease X died because of the disease. But we can certainly say that in the year 2015, for every 100 new cases of disease X, there were 20 deaths reported. In other words, we can say that the numerator is not entirely a part of the denominator. So, death to case ratio is strictly a ratio, NOT a proportion.

We now need to look at the disease Y. In our hypothetical example, we assumed that the same country in the same year had 500 new cases of disease Y and death of 150 patients out of those who were suffering from it.

$$\text{Death to Case Ratio (Disease Y)} = \frac{150 \text{ (deaths due to disease Y in the year 2015)}}{500 \text{ (new cases of disease Y reported in 2015)}}$$

$$\text{Death to Case Ratio (Disease Y)} = \frac{150}{500} \times 100 = 30 \text{ deaths for every 100 new cases}$$

When we compare the death to case ratio for disease X with that for disease Y what we realize is, although the absolute number of deaths are lesser for disease Y, its death to case ratio is higher than that for disease X. it explains the importance of denominator.

Case-Fatality Rate

We have seen above in the discussion on death to case ratio that some of the deaths in a given year occurred in cases which belong to the preceding year. If we confine the numerator also to deaths which occurred among incident cases only for the particular year, then we get 'Case Fatality Rate' which is a measure of the severity of a disease. The case-fatality rate is defined as the proportion of cases of a specified disease or condition which are fatal within a specified time.[27] Formula for calculation will make it more clear-

$$\text{Case-fatality Rate} = \frac{\text{Number of deaths of cases of a given disease out of incident cases that occurred in a given period}}{\text{Total number of incident cases of the disease in the same period.}} \times 10^n$$

From the above formula, what we understand is that the numerator, i.e., number of deaths is strictly a part of the denominator here, i.e., the total number of incident cases. Therefore, Case-fatality rate is a proportion in the true sense and not a ratio. In other words, **case-fatality rate** is the proportion of persons with the disease who die from it in a given period.[1]

Death to Case Ratio and Case Fatality Rate- Principle Difference

*Death to case ratio indicates towards two points, one, is the number of deaths due to some disease in a given period and two, **total prevalent cases** of that disease in the same period. As against this, the case fatality rate tells us how many deaths are occurring due to a disease in a given period out of its **total incident cases** in the same period.*

Age Specific Mortality Rate

Merely knowing how many persons are dying from a specific disease does not fulfill the public health purpose. It is necessary to have an understanding of the specific age group that is worst affected by the fatality of a disease. You must have read or heard statements like 'over last decade the trends of mortality due to cardiovascular diseases have changed, there is an increase in the mortality in the age group 20-40 years in comparison to a previous decade'. What does it tell us? It tells us that to understand trends in specific age groups we need to know mortality for various age brackets that are significant. We can do this by knowing age-specific mortality rates. Let's look at the formula;

$$\text{Age Specific Mortality Rate (In a given age group)} = \frac{\text{Total number of deaths in the given age group in given period}}{\text{Total number of persons in the given age group in mid-point of the period}} \times 10^n$$

In the formula above, the multiplication factor 10^n indicates that we can express this rate for 1000, 10000 or 100000 population as per our requirements. However, we should not forget specifying the population unit size while expressing it.

Some other important age-specific mortality rate examples are discussed in following paragraphs.

Infant Mortality Rate (IMR)

Infant mortality rate, an example of age specific mortality rate, is one of the key development indicators, regarded as a measure of the effectiveness of preventive, promotive and curative services that are focussed on child survival. As the name implies, it is referring to a specific age i.e. infancy or age bracket from birth up to the first birthday.

For a defined period, if we try to see how many children, less than one year of age, are dying for every 1000 live births then it gives us the infant mortality rate for that particular period. The time-period for estimating IMR is one year. As per the standard definition, infant mortality rate is the probability of a child born in a specific year or period, dying before reaching the age of one.[28, 29] Let us look at the formula-

$$Infant\ Mortality\ Rate = \frac{Number\ of\ deaths\ among\ children\ under\ one\ year\ of\ age\ in\ a\ specified\ period}{Total\ number\ of\ live\ births\ in\ the\ same\ period} \times 1000$$

For the IMR, if we have a close look at the formula above, then we can understand that the numerator in this formula is not entirely a part of the denominator. Does it sound confusing? Let's simplify this further. All deaths that are factored into the numerator are not out of the total live births that have taken place in the specified year (time period). Some of the children less than one year of age, who died in the given year, must have been born in the preceding year. Therefore, we can say that IMR is a ratio and NOT a proportion.

Neonatal Mortality Rate

This is another important indicator of child survival situation. As per the definition, neonatal mortality rate is the number of deaths during the first 28 completed days of life, per 1 000 live births in a given year or period.[28, 29] Let's see how to calculate it-

$$Neonatal\ Mortality\ Rate = \frac{Number\ of\ deaths\ among\ neonates\ from\ birth\ up\ to\ (but\ not\ including)\ 28^{th}\ day\ of\ life\ in\ a\ specified\ period}{Total\ number\ of\ live\ births\ in\ the\ same\ period} \times 1000$$

Post-Neonatal Mortality Rate

It indicates mortality among children from age 28 days up to (but not including) 1 year.[1] In other words, post-neonatal mortality is the difference between infant mortality and neonatal mortality.[29] For the calculation of post-neonatal mortality rate, the numerator used is the number of deaths among children of this age group as specified above, during a given period. The denominator is the number of live births during the same period. Like IMR and Neonatal mortality rates, the post-neonatal mortality rate is also expressed per 1,000 live births.

$$\text{Post-Neonatal Mortality Rate} = \frac{\text{Number of deaths among newborns from 28 days of life up to (but not including) 01 year, in a specified period}}{\text{Total number of live births in the same period}} \times 1000$$

Once we have understood the concept of these rates, then referring to table 5 below will help us understand them quickly;

Table 5: Summary of mortality rates among infants

NEONATAL MORTALITY	POST-NEONATAL MORTALITY
Deaths from Birth up to (but not including) 28th day of life- in a given time period- (a year)	Deaths from 28th day up to (but not including) the first birthday –in a given time period (a year)
INFANT MORTALITY	
Deaths from birth up to (but not including) the first birthday • The denominator for all these three indicators is ' total LIVE births that took place in the given time period (defined year). • All these three rates are usually expressed for every 1000 live births that took place in the defined year (i.e. the multiplication factor 10^n is 10^3 i.e.,1000).	

Under-Five Mortality Rate

It gives us an understanding of the situation of entire child survival interventions which extend from pregnancy to early childhood, including preventive, promotive and curative services including immunization, adequate nutrition, care during illness, etc.

By definition, under-five mortality means the total number of children dying in the period from birth up to the 5th birthday, for every 1000 live births. It indicates the probability of a child born in a specific year or period dying before reaching the age of 5 years, if subject to age-specific mortality rates of that period, expressed per 1000 live births.[30,31] All these deaths need to be in a defined time frame, as is the case with other childhood mortality rates that we discussed in preceding paragraphs. Looking at the formula will give us further clarity-

$$\text{Under-5 mortality rate} = \frac{\text{Number of deaths of children from birth to 5}^{th}\text{ birthday in a specified period}}{\text{Total number of live births in the same period}} \times 1000$$

Child Mortality Rate

This rate indicates the probability of children dying between exact ages one year and five years, i.e., between 1st birthday and 5th birthday.[31] We can see that the neonatal and postneonatal mortality, and therefore, the infant mortality are not included in the numerator. Child mortality rate is, therefore, a better indicator if we specifically want to look at post-infancy child health situation.[32]

$$\text{Child mortality rate} = \frac{\text{Number of deaths of children between 1}^{st}\text{ and 5}^{th}\text{ birthday in a specified period}}{\text{Total number of live births in the same period}} \times 1000$$

Sex-Specific Mortality Rate

Any of the above mortality rates can be sex-specific either for males or females. To make them so, we need to make sure that both numerator and denominator are limited to that specific sex for which we are calculating the sex-specific mortality.[1] Let's understand it with some examples:

$$\text{Under-5 mortality rate (}\textbf{\textit{girls}}\text{)} = \frac{\textit{Number of deaths of girl children from birth to 5}^{th}\textit{ birthday in a specified time period}}{\textit{Total number of live births of girl children in the the same period}} \times 1000$$

$$\begin{array}{c}\textit{Age Specific Mortality Rate} \\ (\textit{For }\textbf{\textit{women age 30-39 yrs.}}) \end{array} = \frac{\textit{Total number of }\textbf{deaths of women}\textit{ }\textbf{30-39 years of age}\textit{ in given period}}{\textit{Total number of women in the age group 30-39 years in mid-point of the period specified}} \times 10^n$$

We can make many of these rates double specific. In the above example, we have introduced age specification as well as sex specification for calculating mortality. Along similar lines, if such need arises, we can make calculations for race-specific mortality, occupation-specific mortality so on and so forth. Also, we can further make these rates specific for a particular sex, based on requirements.

Maternal Mortality Ratio

It is the number of deaths during a given period among women while pregnant or within 42 days of termination of pregnancy, irrespective of the duration and the site of the pregnancy, from any cause related to or aggravated by the pregnancy or its management, but not from accidental or incidental causes. Usually, the maternal mortality is expressed per 100,000 live births.[1]

For our basic understanding of the definition at this moment, we should remember that accidental, incidental deaths (or non-obstetric deaths) are those deaths that occur during pregnancy but are not related to it. For example, a death of a woman due to accident while she is pregnant or death due to poisoning etc. For ease of understanding, we will break the definition of maternal mortality into its important constituent segments;

- *Indicating what-* Deaths
- *Among whom-* Women
- *When-* while pregnant, or during childbirth or within 42 days of termination of pregnancy, irrespective of duration and site of pregnancy
- *Why-* from any cause related to or aggravated by the pregnancy or its management
- *Excluding what-* deaths from accidental or incidental causes (non-obstetric deaths)

Each of these segments in the definition is critically important and cannot be ignored in the process of determining maternal mortality. However, to keep the formula simple, we articulate the numerator and denominator in the following way-

$$\text{Maternal Mortality Ratio} = \frac{\text{Number of maternal deaths* in given geography in the given year}}{\text{Total number of live births in the same geography in the same period}} \times 100{,}000$$

Maternal Mortality Rate

It is defined as the number of maternal deaths in a specified period, per 1000 women in the reproductive age group in the given population during the given period.[34]

---

* 'Maternal deaths' in the numerator imply deaths as mentioned in the definition of maternal mortality, i.e., death of women due to any cause related to or aggravated by pregnancy, or its management, during pregnancy or childbirth or within 42 days of termination of pregnancy, irrespective of the site and duration of pregnancy. This excludes incidental or accidental (non-obstetric) causes of death.[33]

BURDEN OF DISEASE-SOME CONCEPTS

A consistent and comparative description of the burden of diseases and injuries and the risk factors that cause them is an important input to health decision-making and planning processes. To ensure availability of reliable information for this purpose, the World Health Organization (WHO) started first Global Burden of Disease (GBD) study in 1990.[35]

The burden of any disease can be judged by different indicators of morbidity and mortality associated with that particular disease. We know that all disease occurrences do not necessarily result in death. Diseases vary widely regarding their ability to cause death, or regarding leaving a residual deficit which can turn a person less productive. There are also variations regarding the sickness spell length. Also, there are huge differences relating to the effectiveness of treatment, cost of treatment and investigations, etc. For some diseases, it is best to focus on prevention because treatment for them is either not available or very costly if available. Some diseases have higher prevalence but cause a less adverse impact on those affected and on the health systems.

In an ideal situation, every individual should live a long life that is healthy and fully productive. Diseases distort this scenario. Some people die before the age they are expected to live up to, while others suffer disability caused due to diseases.

The first GBD 1990 study quantified the health effects of more than 100 diseases and injuries for eight regions of the world in 1990. It generated comprehensive and internally consistent estimates of mortality and morbidity by age, sex, and region. The study also introduced a new metric – the disability-adjusted life-year (DALY) – as a single measure to quantify the burden of diseases, injuries and risk factors. The DALY is based on years of life lost from premature death and years of life lived in less than full health.[35] The WHO supports individual countries to derive estimates at the country level, known as the National Burden of Disease (NBD) estimates, to help them develop country-level plans to reduce the burden of diseases.[35]

In this context, we will try to understand two important concepts, DALYs and QALYs, in the ensuing section:

Disability Adjusted Life Years (DALYs)

To quantify fatal (mortality) and non-fatal outcome of a disease into a single combined summary measure of population health, the concept of DALYs is used. It combines time lived with disability and time lost due to early death in a single metric.

One DALY can be thought of as one lost year of "healthy" life. The sum of these DALYs across the population, or the burden of disease, can be thought of as a measurement of the gap between current health status and an ideal health situation where the entire population lives to an advanced age, free of disease and disability. DALYs for a disease or health condition are calculated as the sum of the Years of Life Lost (YLL) due to premature mortality in the population and the Years Lost due to Disability (YLD) for people living with that disease or health condition or its consequences.[36]

The formula used is;

$$DALYs = YLL + YLD \qquad (37)$$

Let's try to understand this using a simple example. Suppose a man living in a country, where life expectancy for males is 80 years, develops hypertension and subsequently cerebrovascular accident (CVA), resulting in paralysis of left lower limb, at the age of 35 years. The man finally dies due to cardiac failure at the age of 50 years. So, a man who was expected to live a healthy life up to 80 years of age died at the age of 50 years because of hypertension and its complications, which means he lost 30 years of life (YLL) as he died prematurely. From age 35 years to age 50 years (i.e. for 15 years) he was not healthy but had some disability because of the disease and its complications. Before we move further with this example, we need to have basic understanding of disability weights from the next paragraph.

Studies on the Global Burden of Disease are available, which have assigned disability weights to different disease conditions and related complications. Theses disability weights are assigned values between 0 and 1, depending on the severity of the condition. Disability weight 0 implies perfect health (where there is no disability) and 1 implies complete disability (death).

If we multiply the period for which a person was disabled, with the given disability weight then we get the value of DALYs for the years lived with disability (YLD). Let's now refer back to our example of hypertension above. The person in our example suffered from hypertension, CVA and other complications from the age 35 years and continued suffering up to age 50 years when he finally died (**Scenario 1**). So, he suffered for a duration of 15 years. Now, let's assume that the disability weight for CVA and resulting paralysis of the left lower limb is 0.8. The morbidity related YLDs would be:

$$YLD = \text{duration of disability} \times \text{disability weight}$$
$$YLD = 15 \times 0.8 = 12 \text{ DALYs}$$

We already know that DALYs are the sum of YLL and YLD.

In this example, the YLL due to mortality would be;

$$YLL = 80 \text{ (years expected to live)} - 50 \text{(years actually lived)} \times 1$$
$$YLL = 30$$

So, in our example total loss of DALYs would be 30 (YLL due to premature death) + 12 (YLD) = 42 DALYs. Please remember, when the DALYs are actually calculated, some other steps like age weighting and discounting are also involved. *Here, our aim was to present the conceptual clarity about DALYs, hence those processes are not being discussed.*

Please see the graphical illustration (figure 6) of another hypothetical example. No description and details of the medical condition are being mentioned. Please note that the values are different from the above example:

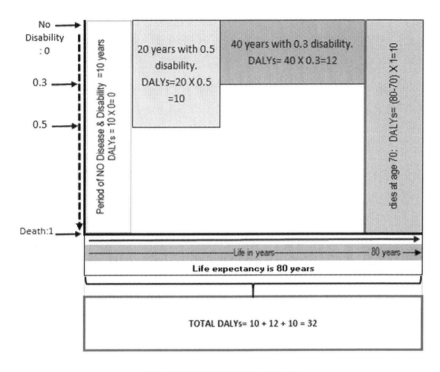

THE GRAPH IS NOT TO SCALE

Figure 6: Illustration Showing Computation of DALYs

The above figure is developed on the basis of presentation in a publication in Norsk Epidemiologi.[38]

There is another point about DALYs which we should try to understand here. We will continue referring back to our example of hypertension and CVA here also. Suppose, with some newer and highly effective medications and lifestyle changes, the patient's blood pressure was perfectly controlled and he was saved from further complications. With treatment, the paralysis which he had developed in left lower limb, improved very well. Physiotherapy helped him restore functionality of his leg to near normal. Only some muscles groups had a residual weakness. Disability weight assigned to this residual condition was 0.3, and the patient survived up to age 70 years with no further improvement or deterioration. Finally, he died at the age 70. **(Scenario 2)**

Let's now look at the DALYs for scenario 2. The individual suffered at age 35 years and had some disability up to 70 years of age, i.e. for a period of 35 years. The disability weight was 0.3 (this is a hypothetical example). So, the DALYs for this morbidity duration and severity would be-

DALYs (morbidity) = 35 (duration) X 0.3 (disability weight) = 10.5

The individual was expected to live up to age 80 years but died prematurely at the age of 70 years. Let's calculate the DALYs for mortality now-

DALYs (mortality) = (80-70) X 1 = 10

Total DALYs (morbidity plus mortality) = 10.5 + 10 = 20.5

Now, we will compare the two scenarios of treatment and find out the differences in total DALYs. Scenario 1 had loss of 42 DALYs, whereas the newer approach, i.e. scenario 2, resulted in the loss of 20.5 DALYs. In other words, we can say 'in scenario 2, where the new treatment approach was applied, we could avert 21.5 DALYs'. Therefore, new treatment approach (scenario 2) is certainly a much better approach in comparison to old approach where the individual died at the age of 50 years. We must note that there are some other factors like age weight and discounting that are involved in the final DALY calculations. Those details are not being discussed here.

Some Uses of DALYs Estimation;

1. DALYs estimation is a common metric for measuring the impact of morbidity and mortality caused by a given disease or condition
2. We can make comparisons of disease burden across different diseases by comparing their impact in terms of loss of DALYs.
3. We can make comparisons between treated and untreated diseases and analyze the benefit of treatment in terms of DALYs averted.
4. By using DALYs, we can also make comparisons between different intervention strategies by seeing how many DALYs are averted when each of these strategies is put into action. For example, prevention strategies versus expansion of treatments.[38]

Quality Adjusted Life Years (QALYs);

DALYs indicate healthy years lost whereas QALYs indicate healthy years gained. In DALYs, we make adjustments for disability whereas, in QALY, adjustments are made for quality of life. In this sense, QALY approach is somewhat opposite to DALYs approach.

In QALYs we assign quality weights to disease conditions which range between 0 and 1, Quality weight 0 meaning death and 1 meaning perfect health.[39] In DALYs, disability weights were also in the same range, but there, 0 means perfect health (no disability) and 1 means full disability (death).[40] In QALY, for a condition of no disease (disease free) the weight would be 1, for less severe conditions that cause a less adverse impact on the quality of life, the weight scores would be little less than 1, like 0.9, 0.8, etc. For conditions causing a more adverse impact on the quality of life, the weight scores will show a larger shift towards 0, like 0.4, 0.3, 0.2, etc.

Now, let's try to understand through an example. Suppose a person, at the age of 17 years, develops some disability which has a quality of life weight of 0.75. He continues with that disability and dies a premature death at the age of 60 years. Assume that the life expectancy is 80 years for men in that geographical area.

Let's try to do some calculations here. QALYs lived by that person before he gets the disability, i.e., at 17 years, would be;

= 1 *(no disability)* X 17 *(years for which the individual lived quality life)*
= *17 QALYS*

QALYs lived by the person during the period when he had the disability would be the product of quality weight for the disabling condition and period for which the person had that condition-

=0.75 *(quality weight)* X 43 *(from 17 years to 60 years)*
=*32.25 QALYs*

So, in his life of 60 years that person has lived 17 + 32.25 = 49.25 Quality Adjusted Life Years. Refer to the graphical illustration of this calculation in the illustration below (figure 7);

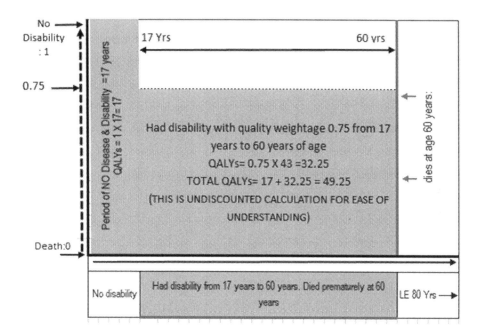

Figure 7: illustration showing computation of QALYs

The above figure is developed on the basis of presentation in a publication in Norsk Epidemiologi.[38]

Let's imagine a situation where some newer treatment extended the life of the patient by ten years, but the degree of disability and the qualitative weight remained the same. Now, what will happen to the QALYs? Everything remains the same except prolongation of life by ten years. So, the QALYs gained with extension of life by ten years would be-

Additional QALYs = quality weightage X extension of life
= 0.75 X 10 = 7.5 *QALYs* gained with the extension of life by ten years with the same disability and the same quality weight, i.e., 0.75.

DALYs and QALY approach is an important concept used in cost-effectiveness analysis for health economics applied to evaluate different interventions. Every student of public health needs to have conceptual clarity on this.

 Points to Remember

- Definitions of incidence and prevalence, interrelation between them.
- How to calculate incidence and prevalence.
- What is crude death rate.
- What is cause-specific death rate.
- What is proportional mortality.
- Difference between death to case ratio and proportional mortality ratio.
- What is age-specific mortality.
- Understand neonatal, infant, perinatal, child and under-five mortality rates.
- Difference between maternal mortality rate and ratio.
- Burden of disease concept, DALYs and QALYs.

CHAPTER

5

Basic Approaches and Methods in Epidemiology

Learning Objectives

- ❖ Get an idea about what different kinds of studies epidemiologists conduct.
- ❖ understand why do they need descriptive epidemiological methods.
- ❖ learn about the broad purpose an analytical (or observational) epidemiologic method serves.
- ❖ know what do epidemiologists basically do in experimental epidemiological methods.

THE WORK EPIDEMIOLOGISTS DO

The practice of epidemiology is based on a methodical approach to study diseases or health-related events. We also need to understand what work an epidemiologist does. Let's see the kind of activities the epidemiologists carryout:

- Find the number of disease cases or health events (the disease burden).
- Understand what is the person, place, and time distribution of these diseases.
- Determine appropriate denominators so that with the application of some specific formula, relevant rates can be calculated.
- Make a comparison between different population groups using these rates.
- Analyze the factors that contribute towards causation of diseases or health-related events.
- Develop some experimental models and try to study the disease occurrence and its association with other possible factors.

If you want to find the numbers of anything, then you must be very clear in your head about what to count. If you are supposed to count pigeons, then you should know what does a pigeon look like. You should not include other birds, which resemble pigeon, in that count. Otherwise, you will get a wrong picture about the total number of pigeons.

Similarly, it is important to have clarity about the disease or health events before trying to determine their numbers. Here we see the importance of formulating a clear and standard case definition. Why clear? Because it can be easily understood without any ambiguity. Why standard? Because every member of the team of epidemiologists should follow the same definition if they all are working to study the same disease or health event.

Once the numbers of cases are found out (using a standard case definition), the next task is to study the distribution of these cases. Distribution can be in terms of persons involved, places affected or the time when such occurrence is commonly seen.

The next logical step will be to see if the occurrence of the particular disease/health event under study is more than what we usually expect. How can we do that? By comparing rates, isn't it? So, calculation of rates of occurrence and making a comparison of different population groups, places or time periods under study is critically important. Otherwise, in the absence of such comparisons how would it be possible for epidemiologists to draw conclusions like 'high rates of occurrence (of a given disease] are noted in tribal adolescent population in two districts of Madhya Pradesh around the end of harvesting season'?

Once we know the numbers and distribution, then we would want to understand what is that which is causing this increased occurrence.

Sometimes, as in case of newly emerging diseases, the epidemiologists do not have the understanding of factors and their association with disease causation. To understand such associations, they develop some experimental models and try to find out all those details.

Now, we are clear that there are different, yet interconnected categories of work that epidemiologists perform. Accordingly, we group these tasks in specific branches of epidemiology. These are descriptive epidemiology, observational or analytical epidemiology, and experimental epidemiology. Before going into details of these methods in subsequent chapters, we will try here to get some clarity about them. To understand it better, you will have to refer back to the section on 'the work epidemiologists do', on the previous page, and figure out which of the points mentioned there fit into different epidemiological methods briefly mentioned below;

BRIEF INTRODUCTION TO EPIDEMIOLOGICAL METHODS

Descriptive epidemiological methods: As the name suggests these methods help us in describing the case burden (number of cases). We come to know how these cases are distributed over the defined geography. We can see if there is any specific pattern which shows that some specific category of people is worst affected (like children, teenage girls, tribal men, persons with sedentary life-style, newly married women, pregnant women of age less than 20 years, or women above 45 years of age, etc). Or, is there any specific season or time of the year when the disease occurs (like peak traffic hours, weekends, winter months, post-monsoon months etc.). After this, we can determine appropriate rates or proportions related to the disease under study. Epidemiologists propose a certain hypothesis based on findings from the descriptive studies.[1]

Observational/Analytical epidemiological methods: In order to understand in what way the disease in question is occurring at higher rates in the population under study, we need to make comparisons with other population groups. Also, we require understanding on which all factors could have played a role in disease causation. For extracting all such information, observational/analytical epidemiological studies are needed. Based on the findings of these studies, hypotheses proposed by descriptive studies around causation are verified.[1, 5]

Experimental epidemiological methods: In these methods, the investigating epidemiologists, in order to further confirm the cause-effect relationship, do some experimenting with the factors that are suspected or thought to have played a role in the causation of the disease under study. Based on the evidence from these experimental studies, some key attributes of a cause-effect relationship between the factor under study and the disease outcome are verified. All these are done through experimental epidemiology methods.[5]

In subsequent chapters, we will look into details of descriptive, observational/analytical and experimental epidemiologic methods.

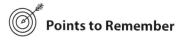
Points to Remember

- ❖ Different categories of work done by epidemiologists.
- ❖ Utility of descriptive details that are generated by descriptive epidemiological methods.
- ❖ Basic approach in analytical epidemiologic methods and the kind of inference drawn out of such findings.
- ❖ Approach and purpose of experimental epidemiologic methods.

CHAPTER

6

Descriptive Epidemiology

Learning Objectives

- Understand the broad objective of descriptive epidemiologic methods.
- Know the steps that are involved in a descriptive epidemiologic study.
- Understand how case definition heps us in descriptive methods.
- Understand the concept of place, person and time distribution of diseases.
- Learn basic concepts of approaches to describe magnitude of a disease.
- Know, in what way descriptive methods help us formulate hypothesis.
- Understand the importance of time, place and person distribution details.

As the name suggests, descriptive studies provide us with some description of the disease. This approach involves the study of disease frequency and its distribution by time, place, and person. We also calculate the rates related to the diseases under study and identify if there are any parts/groups of the population which are at higher risk of developing the disease than others. Sometimes, in situations where the association between exposure and disease is clear, the descriptive investigations alone give us all required details which are sufficient enough to plan and implement control measures.[1]

Descriptive studies, like case investigations, generate hypotheses that can be tested with analytic studies.

STEPS INVOLVED IN DESCRIPTIVE STUDIES

A descriptive epidemiological study will have following steps –

1. Defining the study population (characteristics, composition, specific conditions, etc.)
2. Defining the disease (or health-related condition) to be studied
3. Collecting information about the disease in the affected community/population
4. Describing the disease by time, place and person (to understand distribution of disease)
5. Finding the extent to which the disease under study is affecting the population
6. Comparing rates over different periods or places or population groups as relevant
7. Generating aetiological hypothesis

1. Defining Study Population

Descriptive epidemiological studies carry out investigations on populations/sections of population/population groups. Individuals comprise these groups but, the focus of descriptive studies is on the study population as a whole.

In situations where the population is large, a representative sample of the population is taken for study. Suppose a population, to be studied, is a mix of Hindus, Muslims, Sikhs, and Christians. If a sample comprising of Hindus and Muslims is drawn out from this population, then it is not representative of the population to be studied. So, to say, the sample should be representing all characteristics of a population to be representative. For methodologies to determine sample size, you are requested to refer to your textbook on biostatistics.

For defining the study population, epidemiologists need to focus on various characteristics like age, sex, religious groups, cultural practices, specific exposures to the disease-causing environment, etc. Details like educational status, occupation, environmental factors, dietary habits, etc. are also highly relevant, the list is endless. It is important to ensure that not any of the relevant dimension is missed out.

2. Defining Disease Under Study

It is of paramount importance to define disease to be studied in a crystal-clear manner. The epidemiological criteria to define a disease may not appear exactly like the definition of that disease which clinicians follow. In fact, these criteria help us to measure the quantum of disease in the study population. We will try to understand the features of case definition in the section below;

Case Definition

What epidemiologists use is the operational definition of diseases to be studied. These operational definitions should be such that these help us detect the disease in a given community with a degree of accuracy.[1, 5, 41]

Let us take the example of malaria to understand it;

Description:

The first symptoms of malaria (most often fever, chills, sweats, headaches, muscle pains, nausea, and vomiting) are often not specific and are also found in other diseases (such as influenza and other common viral infections).

Likewise, the physical findings are often not specific (elevated temperature, perspiration, tiredness).[42]

In severe malaria (caused by *P. falciparum*), clinical findings (confusion, coma, neurologic focal signs, severe anemia, respiratory difficulties) are more striking and may increase the suspicion index for malaria.[42]

We have different categories for labelling a case. In reference to malaria here are some terms which are important;

Suspected Case:

As suspected case of malaria is defined as the illness suspected by a health worker to be due to malaria, generally on the basis of the presence of fever with or without other symptoms.[43]

Presumed Case:

Case suspected of being malaria that is not confirmed by a diagnostic test.[43]

Laboratory Criteria for Confirmation

- Detection of circulating malaria-specific antigens using rapid diagnostic test (RDT)

  OR

- Detection of species-specific parasite DNA in a sample of peripheral blood using a Polymerase Chain Reaction (PCR) test (approved and validated test methodology).

  OR

- Detection of malaria parasites in thick or thin peripheral blood films, determining the species by morphologic criteria, and calculating the percentage of red blood cells infected by asexual malaria parasites (parasitemia).[42]

Confirmed Case:

Malaria case (or infection) in which the parasite has been detected in a diagnostic test, i.e., microscopy, a rapid diagnostic test or a molecular diagnostic test.[43]

In the definitions given above, it becomes clear that the epidemiological investigations need to be as precise as possible, not leaving any chance of missing even a single suspected case. It is not always possible to confirm all detected cases by laboratory investigations in the field itself. Some of the suspected cases, when subjected to laboratory testing for confirmation may turn out to be non-malaria cases. It is important for the epidemiologists to develop a definition that helps them pick up a case even on slightest of suspicion. Also, such definitions are the operational definitions which are acceptable ones and can be applied to a large number of people with a degree of accuracy.

In reference to malaria, for epidemiological investigations purposes, investigators would focus on two criteria, i.e., suspected cases of fever and confirmation with laboratory diagnosis.

Now, let us try to look at one of the definitions of malaria that is used for ***clinical purposes;***

Malaria is an illness with fever as its cardinal symptom. It can be intermittent with or without periodicity or continuous. Many cases have chills and rigors. The fever is often accompanied by a headache, myalgia, arthralgia, anorexia, nausea, and vomiting. The symptoms of malaria can be non-specific and mimic other diseases like viral infections, enteric fever, etc. Malaria should be suspected in patients residing in endemic areas or who have recently visited the endemic area and presenting with above symptoms.[44]

Malaria is known to mimic the signs and symptoms of many common infectious diseases, the other causes of fever should also be suspected and investigated in the presence of manifestations like running nose, cough and other signs of respiratory infection, diarrhoea/dysentery, burning micturition and/or lower abdominal pain, skin rash/infections, abscess, painful swelling of joints, ear discharge, lymphadenopathy, etc..[44] However, in reference to malaria, all clinical cases are treated as confirmed when the laboratory investigations indicate so.

Try understanding the difference between these two categories of definitions, one which is used for epidemiological purposes and the other one that is used for clinical purposes. This will further clarify our concept.

You must have noticed that the case definitions that epidemiologists use are based on simple and precise criteria. For investigating any disease, epidemiologists follow the epidemiological case definition that is developed for investigation purposes.

3. Describing the Disease By Place, Person and Time

Describing the occurrence and distribution of any disease is vital for planning prevention and control measures. Therefore, it is important to give a complete picture as to show how a given disease is occurring in a population and what is its distribution pattern. Any descriptive epidemiological study, which is also the first phase of any epidemiological investigation, focusses on descriptive information in terms of time, place and persons involved. Let's try to understand it further-

Place

Imagine the first breaking news (imaginary) about a disease outbreak on a television news channel. How does it appear?

> *"Four hundred cases of a food poisoning have been reported from Dharavi, Mumbai, which is the largest urban slum settlement of Asia."*

Will it make any sense or impact if it appears as presented below?

> *"Four hundred cases of a food poisoning have been reported."*

It sounds totally senseless if it does not tell us about the place of occurrence. Similarly, place distribution details are critically important for epidemiological investigations.

Persons

Let us look again at the above example and try to make it more useful. Here is the improved statement;

> *"One hundred cases of a food poisoning have been reported from Dharavi, Mumbai, which is the largest urban slum settlement in Asia. All those who suffered had their dinner at a wedding reception in the*

> *same locality. Affected persons include 29 women, 33 men, 21 children between 5 and 10 years of age and 17 adolescents. All of them had a common non-vegetarian preparation which was served at the dinner. Those who had only vegetarian food are unaffected."*

Obviously, it is making more sense with person details included. Epidemiological investigations detail out further information about the affected persons, such as age brackets, sex distribution, etc.

Time

Let's try to think how to reinforce the above example in order to extract some more useful information. It is not possible to know from the above statement when did this episode occur. Time of occurrence is critical and helps us decide the urgency which should be applied in launching the control measures to put a check on the disease outbreak. At present, the above example leaves us clueless in this regard. Did it happen last month, or last week or a few days back? Nothing is clear. Below is the more informative version-

> *"One hundred cases of a food poisoning have been reported* **last night** *from Dharavi, Mumbai, which is the largest urban slum settlement in Asia. All those who suffered had their dinner at a wedding reception in the same locality. Affected persons include 29 women, 33 men, 21 children and 17 adolescents. All of them had non-vegetarian preparations. Those who had only vegetarian food are unaffected.* **All persons who had non-vegetarian preparation started developing severe symptoms by midnight and early morning of today, i.e., 14th January 2018.**"

Now, we get a sense of time in the above statement, which is very useful to the health authorities for planning prevention, control, and treatment.

4. Finding the Extent to Which the Disease Under Study is Affecting the Population

We have seen in the preceding chapter that incidence and prevalence are two important measures of disease frequency. There are various rates and ratios which can be applied to study the disease occurrence, besides incidence and prevalence. We have explained these in the chapter on the measurement of morbidity and mortality.

The terms incidence and prevalence have been explained in chapter No. 04, and therefore, the basics are not being explained here again.

However, we will briefly discuss cross-sectional and longitudinal studies here as these are important means of estimating disease magnitude in their simplest designs.

1. Cross-Sectional Study:

Cross-sectional surveys are studies aimed at determining the frequency (or level) of a particular attribute, such as a specific exposure, disease or any other health-related event, in a defined population at a *particular point in time*.[45]

At any point of time, in a population, if we want to know the caseload of a particular disease then we will have to collect information from individuals or screen that population with basic screening tests, whichever is relevant. Through this, we will come to know about the total number of cases of that particular disease in the population. It will include both new and old cases. This is the simplest form of epidemiological studies and is also known prevalence study. A cross-sectional study measures the prevalence of health outcomes or determinants of health, or both, in a population at a point in time or over a short period.[46] Generally, for conducting cross-sectional studies, a representative sample of the population is taken, and the findings from a study of such a sample are extrapolated to a larger population, provided that the sample which was taken is representative.

Since Cross-sectional studies are conducted at a given point, they do not take into account the time factor (such as the duration of exposure) associated with exposure resulting in a particular disease condition. Therefore, these studies provide little information about the natural history of diseases or pattern of new cases (incidence). However, some information about association with risk factors can be gathered. For example, if we are conducting a cross-sectional study on chronic bronchitis and we ask the

Descriptive Epidemiology

respondents some questions about smoking-like 'do you smoke'? 'If yes, then how many cigarettes a day?' 'Since how long have you been smoking?' etc. This information will help us understand the association of chronic bronchitis with cigarette smoking.

In an outbreak of a disease, it is the cross-sectional approach that helps us quickly determine the magnitude of the problem. To understand the health profile of a large population, generally, a cross-sectional study approach is followed. For example, in India and many other countries of the world, governments conduct periodical demographic and health surveys. The findings of these surveys are used for formulating national health policy. Since these surveys are repeated at fixed time intervals, they are also useful in assessing trends of specific demographic and health parameters (refer box 1 below).

Box 1
Demographic and health surveys are important ways of assessing health situation in a population. In India, the most important of such surveys is the National Family Health Survey (NFHS). Till date, four rounds of NFHS have been carried out, and the fifth one is planned for the year 2017-18. The latest one, NFHS-4, was conducted in the year 2015-16. NFHS provides estimates on key health and family welfare indicators related to women, men and children. Only those women and men in the reproductive age group, i.e., women 15-49 years and men 15-54 years of age are covered.
Cross-sectional methodology in NFHS provides updates on key population, health and nutrition indicators, including prevalence of HIV, anemia, high blood pressure, elevated blood glucose levels etc. The survey also covers a range of health-related issues, including fertility, infant and child mortality, maternal and child health, perinatal mortality, adolescent reproductive health, high-risk sexual behavior, safe injections, tuberculosis, and malaria, non-communicable diseases, domestic violence, HIV knowledge, and attitudes toward people living with HIV. The information enables the government of India to monitor and evaluate policies and programs related to population, health, nutrition, and HIV/AIDS.[47]

Advantages of Cross-Sectional Studies

> They are easier to conduct than other individual-based studies because no follow-up is required.

- They provide a good picture of the healthcare needs of the population at a particular point in time.
- They can be used to investigate multiple exposures and multiple outcomes.[45]

Disadvantages of Cross-Sectional Studies

- Being based on prevalent (existing) rather than incident (new) cases, they are of limited value to investigate etiological relationships.
- They are not useful for investigating rare diseases or diseases of short duration.
- They are not suitable to investigate rare exposures.
- With cross-sectional studies, establishing the time sequence of events is difficult.[45]

2. Longitudinal Studies:

In longitudinal studies, selected subjects are followed over time with either continuous or intermittent (at pre-decided intervals) monitoring of exposure to the risk factors or health outcomes. Sometimes, these studies go on for decades and at times, these studies can be very brief, conducted over a period of a few weeks or months. As the individual subjects, enrolled for the study in the beginning, are to be tracked for the entire period, some complexities are unavoidable. For example, some subjects might be lost because of mortality or other reasons.

Most longitudinal studies observe associations between exposure to known or suspected causes and subsequent morbidity or mortality. In the simplest design, a sample or cohort of subjects exposed to a risk factor is identified along with a sample of unexposed controls. The two groups are then followed up prospectively, and the incidence of disease in each is measured. By comparing the incidence rates, attributable and relative risks can be estimated. Longitudinal studies are also known as prospective cohort studies.[48]

These studies, however, require a large number of subjects and a long period of follow up to assess whether the event of interest has occurred. This makes longitudinal studies very expensive to conduct. High chances of subjects getting lost to follow up, due to the need of following them up over a long period, is the main drawback of longitudinal studies.[49]

Longitudinal studies serve descriptive as well as analytical purpose. From the analytical viewpoint, these studies are included under analytical methods, with nomenclature 'cohort studies'. For details, please refer to sections on cohort studies given in the chapter on analytical epidemiologic methods.

5. Comparing Rates Over Different Periods or Places or Population Groups

Descriptive epidemiological study findings (time, person and place distribution) help us compare disease magnitudes between periods (e.g., winter months with summer months), between places (example- the incidence of influenza in Delhi and Srinagar) or between persons (example- the prevalence of anaemia in men compared with women). This comparison also guides us in drawing hypothesis that tries to explain the difference between the rates of occurrence of a particular disease between places, groups of persons or over different time periods. When you go through the section on 'usefulness of time, person and place details' given in this chapter, you will find suitable examples to understand this further.

6. Generating Etiologic Hypothesis

An etiological hypothesis is a statement, developed on the basis of available scientific evidence, which can be tested through appropriate research methods, to understand and define the relationship between two or more variables. One of these variables is independent which occurs first (exposure), and the other one is the dependent variable, which is the outcome. Hypothesis statement, so developed, is framed to find answers to the research questions about a particular relationship between these two types of variables.

Many a times epidemiologists in an unbiased way, assume that there is no effect of the independent variable on the outcome. Such an assumption is known as 'null hypothesis.' Etiological hypotheses get refuted or disproved many times, and that situation also provides answers to research questions or gives some important clues to help further probing.

A good etiologic hypothesis should always have the following characteristics:

- It is based on scientific assumptions that are derived from the existing knowledge or observations.
- The hypothesis should include a clear definition of the exposure(s) and outcome(s) of interest.[45]
- The etiological hypothesis is linked to the research question in such a way that it tries to find answers to it.
- It should always be a simple and unambiguous statement.
- The hypothesis should always be a testable statement; a statement that can be tested through appropriate epidemiological methods.

An etiologic hypothesis is highly valuable as it gives direction to the research and helps researchers in staying focused to find answers to the research question.

Descriptive epidemiologic methods provide highly important leads to epidemiologists for developing an etiologic hypothesis. If any disease occurrence is described in terms of person, place and time distribution and no thought is given to the probabilities of etiology then the whole purpose of doing descriptive epidemiological investigation would not be met. The question that arises is- how do epidemiologists generate the etiological hypothesis? In order to do this a great amount of thinking, based on available scientific evidence and observations of descriptive epidemiologic methods, goes into all possibilities and then the most relevant, evidence-driven, simple and testable hypothesis is generated.

There are many sets of information generated from the descriptive epidemiological studies that are used as guiding points in generating a hypothesis. Let's use a simple example to understand it. If a particular febrile illness is reported from an area having plenty of mosquitoes and the most affected persons are in the houses not using any protection measures like repellents and mosquito nets, then there is a possibility that the illness in reference can be a disease transmitted by mosquitoes. Also, the incidence is observed to increase soon after the months when mosquito breeding takes place. Such information can help us form a hypothesis which can be tested further by detailed analysis.

Another example- if a respiratory infection is reported which has affected individuals residing in small houses having poor ventilation. Once a household has an initial case, then other individuals also started getting affected within a period of 7-10 days. First affected were the members sleeping together. This illness particularly peaked during winter months. This information hints at the fact that the causative agent is spreading through close contact, probably through droplets or through fomites. It can be a pathogenic organism that grows at lower environmental temperatures. All such points are valuable in formulating the hypothesis of disease causation.

It is important to remember that sometimes (rather, most of the times) having discussions with persons affected by the illness, their close friends, and relatives, co-workers can give us valuable clues that will help develop an appropriate hypothesis of causation. Similarly, the healthcare persons can give us some valuable information like non-availability of a particular chemoprophylactic drug, for more than 1 year, which was supposed to be given to protect the people residing in a high-risk area for a particular disease, or vaccines which were supposed to be kept in cold chain were actually kept at room temperature for a week and then administered to the children. Such information is valuable and should be used in drawing inferences for generating a hypothesis.

Ideally, a hypothesis formulated should try to justify the reasons for a particular group of people getting affected. It should also tell us why particular geography is involved, is there any reason that is inherent to the socio-cultural practices of the community, are there any other environmental or genetic factors responsible, is there any linkage with health service delivery (or lack of it). Also, the probable routes of transmission (if it is an infectious disease), probable reservoir, any vector involved, etc. are some valuable points that a proposed hypothesis should try to include. In case of non-communicable diseases, individual behaviors and lifestyle, environmental factors, social, cultural factors can give us an important clue for generating the aetiological hypothesis.

It must be remembered that generating a well-founded hypothesis is important. An epidemiological investigation team should carefully examine the hypothesis and try to corroborate it with all available environmental, behavioral, demographic or laboratory indications that are available. If it is generated without using the complete available evidence or clues, then the analytical study based on such hypothesis may not yield conclusive evidence.

TIME, PERSON AND PLACE DETAILS AND THEIR USE

We will see some more examples here, which give us a clear understanding of the importance of time, person and place details.

Time Distribution

Weekly trends and proportion of annual numbers of positive influenza cases, by epidemiologic week and influenza type, in Srinagar (Graph A) and New Delhi (Graph -B), India, 2011–2012 are shown below. Clear seasonal peaks are seen in January–March for Srinagar and in July and September for New Delhi.[50]

Descriptive Epidemiology

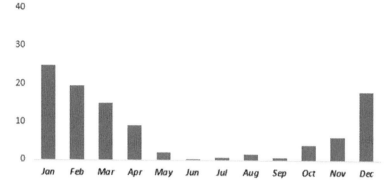

Graph A; Srinagar

Figure 8: Graph showing seasonal trend of influenza cases in Srinagar (produced using indicative percentage based on the study by Parvaiz A. Koul, 2014, for highlighting the seasonal trend. Exact percentages do not match)

Credit: Parvaiz A. Koul[50]

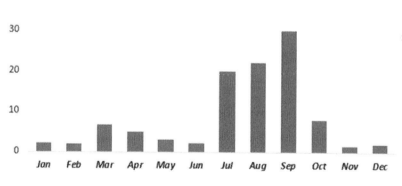

Graph B: Delhi

Figure 9: Graph showing seasonal trend of influenza cases in Delhi (produced using indicative percentage based on the study by Parvaiz A. Koul, 2014, for highlighting the seasonal trend. Exact percentages do not match)

Credit: Parvaiz A. Koul[50]

In the above graphs of influenza cases in two cities of India (figure 8 & 9), we see that there is a clear seasonal trend that can be identified. This is an example of time distribution details given by descriptive studies. We can now figure out when to be on high alert to apply brakes on the transmission and when to focus on gearing up preparedness to minimize the impact.

There are following types of key time-related trends noted in different disease outbreaks:

A. Short-Term Fluctuations

There are many factors which do not exist constantly and may influence disease pattern when they operate. For example, if a place suddenly experiences a severe heatwave which is not expected routinely, it may give rise to an increased number of heat exhaustion and heat stroke cases. This is a sudden impact of an external factor which is causing fluctuations. Likewise, if in an urban area a sewage pipeline bursts and contaminates drinking water source accidentally, then we will see an increased number of gastrointestinal infections, at a level which is not routinely expected. There are so many other examples where short-term fluctuations are noted. You are urged to think and list down some more examples for your benefit.

Periodic Fluctuations

There are some diseases which show a periodic fluctuation, with the highest incidence, noted when some external conditions favor rapid growth of the disease-causing organisms, and there is also a favorable environment for the responsible vectors to grow in numbers. For example, in India, we see a rise in cases of diseases like malaria and dengue during and immediately after the rainy season.

We try to group some of these fluctuation trends as below-

i. Seasonal Trend

Many infectious diseases show an increase in the number of cases during specific seasons. Upper respiratory infections have been found to occur more frequently during winter months, gastrointestinal infections more commonly during monsoon and immediate post-monsoon season. By understanding such trends, the health service delivery system can make necessary preparations to control the disease spread and also to provide adequate and prompt treatment to all affected.[1]

ii. Cyclic Trends

As we know that for any infection to establish the transmission in a community, it is essential that there are susceptible individuals present in that population. When the infection spreads to individuals, they start developing immunity against it and as a result further spread gets reduced, as the proportion of susceptible individuals is reduced. We see a further rise in cases only when the herd immunity declines after some time. Hence, we see a typical cyclical trend in such infections. The trend may show an increase over a period of every few months or years. Measles, for example, had been found to follow such trend over a period of 2-3 years in the periods when vaccination coverage was very poor.

B. Secular Trends (Long-term fluctuations)

These are changes in the disease frequency that persist for a longer term over the duration of years or decades. Epidemiologists and healthcare program administrators can use the knowledge about secular trends to understand the direction in which these trends are shifting and study the reasons for such changes. Disease frequencies on declining or increasing pattern serve as valuable information that can guide public health strategies. Understanding past trends also help us predict future incidence of diseases.[1]

Refer to figure 10, which shows the numbers of poliomyelitis cases in India, from the year 1974 to the year 1994.[51] We can easily notice long-term fluctuations here.

Place Distribution

The significance of place distribution becomes clear when we look at the map in figure 11. It shows us estimated incidence rates for Tuberculosis per 100,000 population, in different parts of the world. Even a quick glance can tell us which countries have a higher burden of tuberculosis. So, we can make a comparison between countries (*International comparisons*).[54]

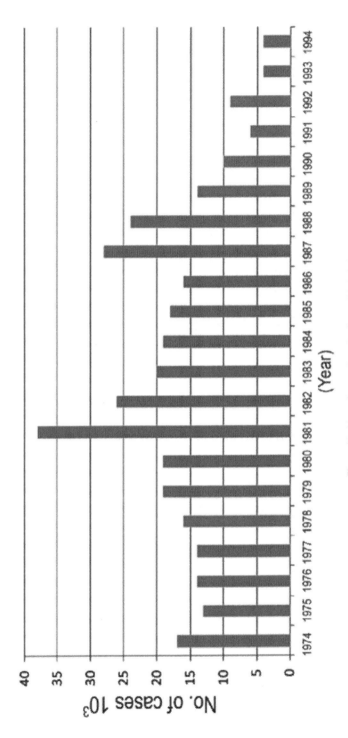

Figure 10: Year-wise number of poliomyelitis in India

Graph Credit: John TJ[52, 53] Retrieved from https://www.ncbi.nlm.nih.gov

Descriptive Epidemiology

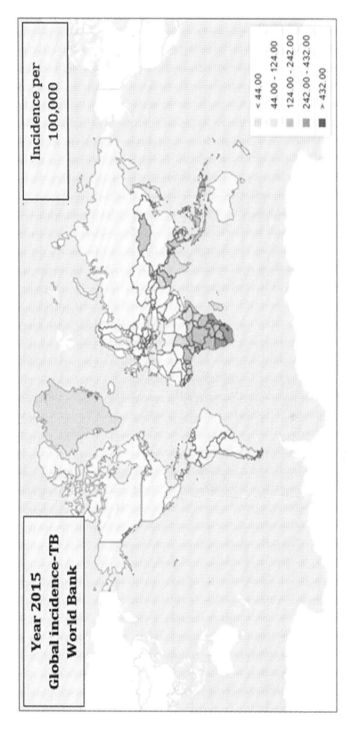

Figure 11: Map Showing Global Incidence of TB

Credit: Taken from the World Bank Data web page https://data.worldbank.org- Incidence of tuberculosis (per 100,000 people) World Health Organization, Global Tuberculosis Report.[54]

Similarly, it is possible to make the comparison within parts of a country and accordingly determine priorities for reinforcing prevention and control measures.

The map below (figure 12) shows one such example in which incidence of Tuberculosis for the year 2014 is shown for different districts of India. *(Inter-district comparison)*. Such comparisons can also be made between the states or provinces to understand the situation.

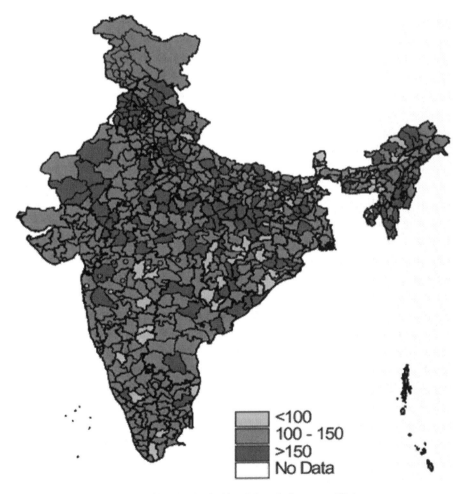

Figure 12: Map showing incident Tuberculosis cases notified per 100,000 population by district of India for the year 2014

Credit: Central TB Division, Ministry of Health &Family Welfare, Govt of India[55]

Descriptive Epidemiology

Such comparisons are needed even within a district and are very helpful for district health authorities to strengthen prevention and control strategies area wise (*local comparisons*). As an example of local comparisons, the map below shows hypothetical percentage case-load of Plasmodium falciparum malaria in a district of India, for the year 2010;

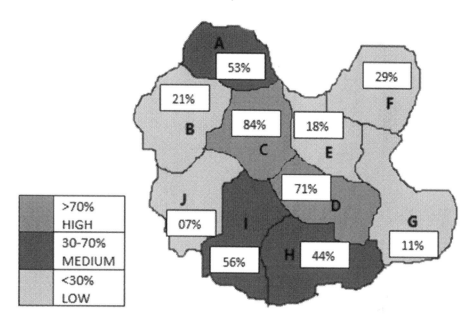

Figure 13: Map showing imaginary caseload of Plasmodium falciparum, in a district of India for the year 2010. Shaded segments of the map represent blocks of the district

Many times, such comparisons are needed in even smaller geographies as these may provide important clues to the investigations. One such example of an investigation of an outbreak of acute hepatitis in Girdhar Nagar locality of Ahmedabad, India, is illustrated below.

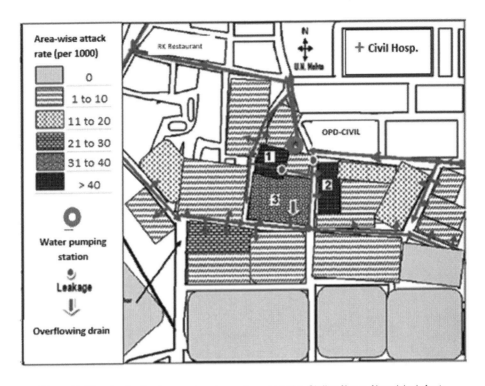

Figure 14: Map showing local comparison in smaller geography- Girdhar Nagar, Ahmedabad, Acute Hepatitis-area wise attack rate (modified for clarity)

Credit: Naresh T Chauhan, Indian J Community Med. 2010 Apr; 35(2): 294–297[56]

Person Distribution

From almost every point of view describing how a disease condition is distributed among persons is important. To decide whether it is promotive, preventive or curative actions that are to be launched in response to a disease outbreak, knowledge about 'who all are affected' and 'who all are at risk' is paramount. Because personal characteristics may influence illness, organization, and analysis of data by "person" may use any of such personal characteristics. These can be inherent characteristics (for example, age, sex, race), biologic characteristics (immune status), acquired characteristics (marital status, educational status), activities (occupation, leisure activities, use of medications/tobacco/drugs), or the conditions under which they live (socioeconomic status, environmental factors, access to medical care).[1]

By looking at the stacked bar diagram below, we can infer that male migrants carry a higher burden of HIV infection in three studied places in India (hypothetical example). Therefore, any strategy formulated against HIV in those three places should have a robust component to cover the risk group 'male migrants'.

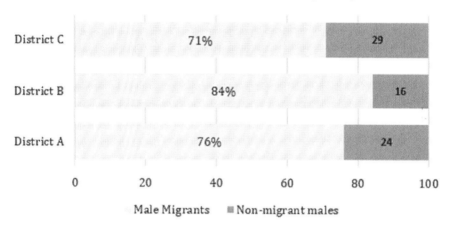

Figure 15: HIV and male migrants-an example to highlight person distribution

Now, let's look at another descriptive report section which gives us information about person distribution. The clustered bar diagram below shows the incidence of Tuberculosis cases in the year 2013 in SEAR (South East Asian Region) countries. We can make out that for almost every age incidence for the year 2013 was higher in males in comparison to females. Also, we can see that there are some age brackets from which the number of cases notified was comparatively higher.[57] It is to be noted that these are merely the numbers, rates are not applied here.

Age and sex distribution of all notified new TB cases in 2013: SEAR member countries

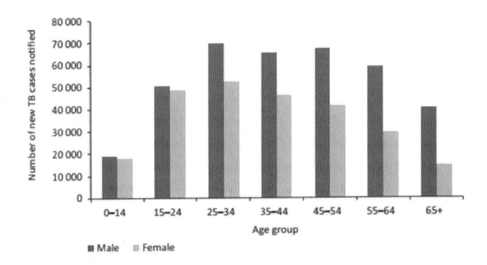

Figure 16: An example showing age and sex wise person distribution
(Includes only data from Bangladesh, Bhutan, Democratic People's Republic of Korea, Indonesia, Maldives, Nepal and Sri Lanka)

Credit: WHO SEAR, Tuberculosis control in South-East Asia Region, Report-2015[58]

One more example could be about children 12-23 months of age who are fully immunized against TB, Polio, Diphtheria, Pertussis, Tetanus, and Measles (primary immunization) in India, as reported by the fourth National Family Health Survey (NFHS-4) conducted in the year 2015-16.

NFHS-4 reported the distribution of fully immunized children 12-23 months of age, based on the educational status of their mothers, caste or tribe group, and wealth quintile to which the family belongs.[59] This gives us an idea about the groups that should be targetted on a priority basis if we want to increase the immunization coverage of children. A careful look at the graph below will clarify it further.

Descriptive Epidemiology

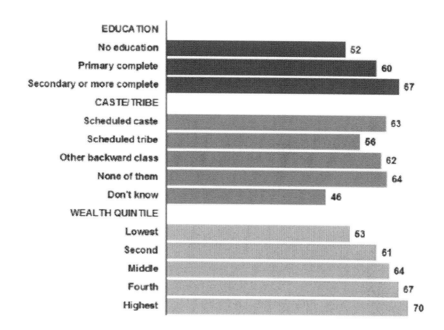

Figure 17: Percentage of children 12-23 months of age who are fully immunized: NFHS-4

Hopefully, you are now able to understand the broad objective as to why we need time, place and person distribution details. Compiling and analyzing data by time, place, and person is desirable for several reasons;

> First, by looking at the data carefully, epidemiologists can make some judgment about it. They can see what the data can or cannot reveal based on the variables available, its limitations (for example, the number of records with missing information for each important variable), and its eccentricities (for example, all cases for some childhood disease are in the range in age from 2 months to 6 years, and there are 11 records showing age 20 years and above).

> Second, the epidemiologists learn the extent and pattern of the public health problem being investigated — which months, which neighborhoods, and which groups of people have the most and least cases.

- Third, the epidemiologists create a detailed description of the health of the population that can be easily communicated with tables, graphs, and maps.
- Fourth, the epidemiologist can identify areas or groups within the population that have high rates of disease. This information, in turn, provides important clues to the causes of the disease, and these clues can be turned into testable hypotheses.[1]

Points to Remember

- Concept of descriptive epidemiological studies
- Steps involved in conducting descriptive epidemiological studies
- Principles of developing a case definition and its components
- Place, person and time distribution-in what way it helps to plan prevention and control activities
- Ways to define magnitude of a disease
- Longitudinal and cross-sectional studies
- Reasons for which we compile data by place, person and time

CHAPTER 7

Analytical Epidemiology

Learning Objectives

- Learn about commonly used analytical epidemiologic methods.
- Understand the conceptual design of case-control studies, learn about right selection of cases and controls, matching them using different approaches.
- Understand the basic approach of analyzing case-control study findings.
- Know what are the merits and demerits of case-control studies.
- Learn about cohort study concept and understand how to do basic analysis on the findings of these studies.
- Get conceptual clarity about Relative Risk, Odds Ratio and Attributable Risk.

We have read in the previous section that a well-founded aetiological hypothesis, generated by any descriptive epidemiological study, needs testing. Such testing is done through analytical epidemiological methods. In the following section, we will try to understand some key analytical methods.

CASE-CONTROL STUDIES

Case-control studies are a comparatively simpler way of studying the causes of diseases and factors contributing to such causation. As the name suggests, in this type of study there are cases (individuals having the disease under study), and there are controls (individuals without the disease). In these studies, the objective of epidemiologists is to compare the degree of occurrence of disease or exposure to factors which may have contributed to the health outcome, i.e., disease. The focus is on selecting cases of the disease under study (persons having the disease at the time of selection). Control group comprises of people having almost identical characteristics as the cases but are free from the disease under study at the time of selection.[1, 5, 60, 61]

Let us take the example of chronic bronchitis and conducting a case-control study on this. First, we select established cases of chronic bronchitis in the case group, using the standard definition of chronic bronchitis. Now, we have to select individuals for the control group. For this task, we will try to identify people with somewhat similar characteristics (example, almost the same age, sex, socio-economic background, environmental conditions and other characteristics), who *do not have chronic bronchitis*. Suppose we are trying to understand the role of smoking in the causation of chronic bronchitis then we will go backward in time and try to understand the smoking habits of cases and controls. Figure 18 represents a basic scheme of a case-control study.

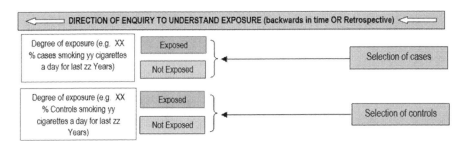

Figure 18: Schematic diagram showing case-control study design

KEY STEPS OF CASE-CONTROL STUDIES

Following are the main steps in any case control study;[5, 45]

1. Selection of Cases

- Cases are selected on the basis of disease and not of exposure
- There should be a standard case definition which is followed throughout the study
- Cases selected should represent all cases in a given population
- Case eligibility criteria are also needed to be defined before beginning selection of cases

2. Selection of Controls

It is important to remember that controls give us a baseline against which we measure the influence of exposure to a particular factor (or factors) in the causation of disease. Therefore, selection of controls must be carried out carefully and they should be closely resembling in key characteristics with the cases, except that they should be free from the disease.[1] Following points must be kept in mind while selecting controls;

- Controls must be free from the disease being studied
- Controls must be from the same population to which cases belong
- They must closely resemble cases in the general demographic characteristics so that we can ensure that the cases and controls are similar.
- Selection of controls (and cases also) must not be influenced by their status of exposure to factors which are being studied.
- Controls can be selected from the household to which a case belongs, or from the neighborhood or the same community.
- For hospital based studies, controls from the same hospital where the cases are admitted can be selected, but these will not be representative

of the general healthy population. Sometimes in hospital-based studies, it becomes unavoidable to have hospitalized controls. In such situation, great care needs to be taken to ensure that their disease, ongoing treatment, and other associated factors do not give us a false judgment about the baseline.

- Studies with a large number of cases can have an equal number of controls but for studies that have a smaller number of cases (20 to 50) epidemiologists often prefer to have multiple controls for each case to get a clear understanding of the baseline by having a better representation of the general population.[5, 45]

3. Matching Cases and Controls

- Select controls in a manner so that they resemble cases as closely as possible. Key individual demographic attributes should be identical or should be as closely matching as possible.[45, 60]

- Matching does not mean that all characters should be 100% identical. For example, for a case who is working as a male agricultural laborer and is of age 51 yrs., 2 months and 03 days, you should not start looking for a control who is exactly of 51 yrs., 2 months and 03 days of age. Rather one should try to find a control who is male, working as an agricultural laborer and preferable of age between 50-53 years.

- Let us now understand a new term 'confounding biases.' **Confounding** is a situation in which the impact of relationship or association between an exposure to a certain factor and outcome of such an exposure gets distorted due to the presence of another variable. Confounding can be of two broad categories; positive confounding and negative confounding. **Positive confounding** is when the observed association shows a stronger exposure-outcome relation in comparison to what actually is. In other words, it is **biased away** from the hypothesis that assumes there is no association between the two, (i.e., null) and **negative confounding**, when the observed association is **biased towards** the null. In other words, negative confounding shows a weaker exposure-outcome association than what it actually is.[5, 62]

> The way we carry out matching influences confounding to a great extent. The characteristics generally chosen for matching are those that are known to be strong *confounders*. Common matching variables are age, sex, and ethnicity but others might be the place of residence, or socioeconomic status etc..[45] To understand linkages between confounding and matching we will take an easy hypothetical example. Suppose there are two hamlets in a village, hamlet A, and hamlet B. These hamlets are identical in most of the socio-cultural and demographic characteristics. Hamlet A has been reporting consistently high rates of gastrointestinal infection among infants. Regular health and nutrition education sessions have been going on in both the hamlets. Health authorities plan to conduct a case-control study to understand what could have led to increased rates of gastrointestinal infections among infants of hamlet A. It was carried out as a project by a team of medical students studying in the department of community medicine. A case-control study was planned, 100 cases were selected from Hamlet A and families having infants were selected as controls from hamlet B. Respondents in the study were mothers who had infants (for hamlet A- mothers of infants who had gastro-intestinal infection episodes in last one year). The study assessed infant feeding awareness and care practices in both these hamlets to understand if there is any exposure to contaminated food or water.

It was found that more than 89% of mothers in the control group were having adequate information about correct infant feeding practices and 78% were practicing the correct methods while feeding infants. As against this, in the case group, only 27% mothers had required information about correct infant feeding practices and only 13% practicing them. This much of difference made investigators relook into all aspects of the study. On scrutinizing the study questionnaire, it was discovered that mothers' education level was not taken into account while matching the controls. Majority of mothers in the case group were either illiterate or had primary level schooling. Whereas, 90% of mothers in the control group had education up to 12th standard and remaining 10% had studied up to graduate level.

This omission of matching educational levels of mothers in case group and control group led to confounding bias in the results. The control group was not representing the universe to which cases were belonging. We hope, now the concept of confounding bias and the need for proper matching of controls with cases is clear.

There are two approaches of matching-one is matching **by groups,** and the other is matching **by pairs.**

a. Matching by Groups:

If we can systematically categorize the case group into suitable strata using key characteristics, then it is a practically better approach to carry out matching of controls by the strata. Stratification can be done by using criteria like age, sex, occupation, literacy, place of inhabitation, income based grouping, or any other relevant criteria which is important for the study. Subsequently, a suitable control group may be selected by carrying out strata-wise matching. Suppose, in a case group for the study on the chronic obstructive pulmonary disease; we find that 20% of cases are rural inhabitants who are living below poverty line. And 70% of them (70% of 20%) are working in cement manufacturing plants (having daily exposure to cement dust), Let us further assume that these two factors may have a bearing on the outcome under study. Now we will have to see that such distribution is available in the control group we select otherwise it will be an improper matching. Improper matching will result in bias (confounding). Therefore, we need to be careful about all such factors while selecting control group.[45]

b. Matching by Pairs:

Matching by pairs implies that for every case you will try to find matching control. This is also known as individual matching.[45] This consumes a lot of time. Suppose, a male accountant of age 50 years, working in a state government public works department, develops lung cancer. This individual gets enrolled as a case in a case-control study to see the role of smoking in the causation of the disease. Now, when we try to find a control for this person then the idea should be to find a person not having lung cancer, doing a similar kind of job, he should be in the same age group (say 49 to 51 years). It would be an impractical approach to look for a control who has the same date, month and year of birth as that of the case, also working in the public works department as an accountant, and so on. This is known as overmatching and is an impractical approach.

4. Understanding Exposure

Now, the investigators of the study will have to understand the exposure to the risk factor under study, both in cases and controls. Exposure of controls to the risk factor gives us a baseline level to make comparisons. Our key risk factor in the example of lung cancer study is *'smoking.'*[5, 45]

For understanding the degree and duration of smoking the most practical way is to administer a questionnaire, that is prepared for finding the exposure, to cases and controls. This requires very simple questions like 'do you smoke (cigarette, bidi, tobacco in pipe)?', 'what was your age when you started smoking?', 'for how many years in total have you been smoking?', 'how many cigarettes/bidis have you been smoking every day?' so on and so forth.

Upon ascertaining exposure to cigarette smoking, we will know that there are some cases and some controls who are exposed to a certain level of smoking whereas there are other cases and controls who are not exposed to it. Cigarette smoking is a known risk factor for lung cancer; this fact is very well established now. But still this example is taken here for two reasons, one, it is a simple and direct example, and the second reason is to give a message to all readers that one should avoid getting into the habit of smoking.

In this study, we need to examine if lung cancer in the majority of our study cases is associated with the long history of cigarette smoking, with a higher number of cigarettes smoked per day, as compared to the control group, which is free of disease. Just to remind, we trace backward over time to understand exposure to risk factors in those who have developed the disease (cases) and in those who are free of disease (controls).

5. Analysing Exposure-Disease Association

In this section, we will familiarize ourselves with two important concepts which are Relative Risk (RR) and Odds Ratio (OR). RR is used in prospective studies (e.g., cohort) while OR is calculated in a case-control (retrospective) studies.[5]

To understand these concepts, we will have to look for two interesting sets of information. First, is the number and proportion of persons among cases who have been exposed to the risk factor for the disease under study. The second is the number and proportion of controls who are exposed to the same risk factor under study.[5, 45]

To understand it, let's take a new example of a study trying to examine the association of alcohol intake with cirrhosis of liver. Assuming that the study enrolled 50 cases who have cirrhosis of liver and 60 matching controls who do not have the disease. Out of 50 cases who have the disease, 45 gave the history of alcohol intake of long standing. For the controls, who do not have cirrhosis of liver, only 10 gave a positive history for alcohol intake of long standing.

Table 6: Cirrhosis of liver and history of alcohol intake

Exposure (Alcohol Intake) *	Cases (With Liver Cirrhosis)	Controls (Without Liver Cirrhosis)
Consuming Alcohol	45 **(a)**	10 **(b)**
Not Consuming Alcohol	5 **(c)**	50 **(d)**
TOTAL	50	60

From the table number 6 above, we can see that there are total 50 cases, out of whom 45 are giving a history of long-standing alcohol intake. So, the

---

* Alcohol intake of more than 5 years duration

proportion of those having liver cirrhosis, reporting alcohol intake (exposure rate among cases) would be:

= (CASES with alcohol intake/total CASES) X 100 (in %)
= 45/(45+5) X 100= 90 %

Similarly, the proportion of controls who have the history of alcohol consumption (exposure rate among controls) would be:

= (CONTROLs with alcohol intake/total CONTROLS) X 100
= 10/(10+50) X 100= 16.66%

This is a big difference, 90% against 16.66%. It looks like there is a strong association between alcohol consumption and cirrhosis of the liver. But, before coming to this conclusion, we will verify the findings statistically. We will first determine the Standard Error (SE) of difference between two proportions:

$$\text{SE of difference between two proportions} = \sqrt{\frac{p_1 q_1}{n_1} + \frac{p_2 q_2}{n_2}}$$

Where,

p_1 = Proportions of **cases** having exposure (long-standing alcohol intake)
q_1 = Proportion of **cases** NOT having exposure (long-standing alcohol intake)
n_1 = Total number of **cases** in the study
p_2 = Proportions of **controls** having exposure (long-standing alcohol intake)
q_2 = Proportion of **controls** NOT having exposure (long-standing alcohol intake)
n_2 = Total number of **controls** in the study

We will now put values into this formula from the table 6 above

In our example of alcohol intake and cirrhosis of the liver, $p_1=90\%$, $q_1=100-90=10\%$ and $n_1=50$. From the set of controls, our $p_2=16.66\%$, $q_2=100-16.66=83.34\%$ and $n_2=60$.

$$\text{SE of difference between two proportions} = \sqrt{\frac{90 \times 10}{50} + \frac{16.66 \times 83.34}{60}}$$

$$= \sqrt{18.00 + 23.14}$$

$$= \sqrt{41.14}$$

SE of difference between two proportions = **6.42**

In our example above, the two proportions are 90% and 16.66%, and the difference between them is 90-16.66=73.34. Had this difference been within 2 SEs (i.e., 6.42 + 6.42= 12.84) then we could have taken this difference as occurring by chance, But, here the difference is much more than even thrice of SE as calculated above. So, we can conclude that this difference is statistically highly significant and there is an association between alcohol consumption and cirrhosis of the liver as revealed in our study. We can also perform Chi-square test to check whether the difference is significant or not (*you will have to refer to your textbook on biostatistics to understand more of these statistical methods*).

Another important analytical step is to estimate the risk of getting the disease in the exposed study population. We will get a sense of it if we compare disease occurrence among those who are exposed to the risk factor with that among those who are not exposed to the risk factor. Let's apply this to our example. In table 6, we see that 45 cases and 10 controls had the exposure to the risk factor, a total of 55 individuals. So, the occurrence of disease among exposed is –

$$45/(45+10)$$

Whereas in those who are not exposed, the occurrence is-
$$5/(5+50)$$

Now let's compare them to get the *relative risk*

$$= \frac{45/(45+10)}{5/(5+50)}$$
$$= \frac{0.8182}{0.0909}$$
$$= 9$$

Based on our study sample we can say that the risk of cirrhosis of the liver was found to be 9 times more among those who have a history of long-standing alcohol intake, in comparison to those who do not have such a history.

What we have calculated above is known as *Relative Risk* or *Risk Ratio*. Relative Risk or Risk Ratio is defined as the ratio between the incidence of disease among exposed and the incidence among those who are not exposed (to the risk factor in reference). But, we know that in our hypothetical example, the sample drawn is small and is not the true extract from the general population. Imagine the situation if we had screened the population from a given geography to detect cases of cirrhosis of Liver and enquired them for exposure. Under such situation, the estimated relative risk between exposed and non-exposed would have been of validity to be applied to the entire population. In this scenario, we have the 'at risk population denominator' factored in the calculations as we screened the entire population in that area.

Alternatively, if we follow those who are exposed to the risk factor over time and observe how many of them develop the disease, as we do in cohort studies, we can arrive at precise relative risk estimates.

Odds Ratio

This is another measure of association, which is most commonly used in analyzing case-control study results. As we know, the word 'odds' means 'likelihood' or chances of something happening or not happening. Odds ratio shows if there is an increased likelihood of getting the disease on exposure to the factor, or the chances of getting the disease are reduced on exposure, or exposure to the factor does not influence the outcome, i.e., disease.

In Odds ratio, we compare odds (likelihood) of developing a disease for exposed with odds of disease for those who are not exposed to the suspected risk factor.[63]

Let's look at table 06 above again and use the numbers to calculate Odds Ratio for the study observations.

Odds (likelihood) of disease among exposed persons would be-

$$= \frac{a/(a+b)}{b/(a+b)} = a/b$$

Odds of disease among those who are not exposed would be-

$$= \frac{c/(c+d)}{d/(c+d)} = c/d$$

Odds Ratio (OR) is the ratio of the probability of outcome (disease) among exposed and outcome among non-exposed. So, the OR for our study example in table 06 above would be-

$$= a/b \div c/d$$
$$= ad/bc$$

In the formula for OR that we arrived at above, there is a cross multiplication of diagonally opposite cells in our table (a multiplied with d, b multiplied with c). Hence, OR is sometimes referred as **Cross Product Ratio** also. Now, let's put the values from table 6 into this formula and calculate OR-

$$= (45 \times 50) \div (10 \times 5)$$
$$= 2250 \div 50$$

Odds Ratio $\quad\quad = 45$

The value of Odds Ratio is high here as we have taken a hypothetical example showing a high rate of cirrhosis among alcoholics. The rate we have taken is much higher than what is reported by various medical research studies. This was purely to explain the basics of Odds Ratio.

Odds Ratio, as obtained in the example above, indicates there is a high association of prolonged and excessive alcohol intake with cirrhosis of liver. Those who consume excess alcohol *(even this excess level and prolonged time should be defined before we begin the study)* for a prolonged time are 45 times more likely (probability) to get the disease in comparison to those who do not have exposure to alcohol intake of the same degree and duration.

We have calculated RR and OR from the same data set given in table 6. The difference between values should not confuse us. As a rule, when an event or outcome is rare (less than 10%) then OR and RR values are closer to each other. However, when an event or outcome is common, i.e., observed in more than 10% in the unexposed group, the OR will be much higher than the RR, as we are noticing in our example above.

It would be incorrect to make a statement on the risk of cirrhosis of liver associated with excessive and prolonged alcohol intake, based on a single measure of OR derived in our example. The OR value derived here, is based on a study of 50 cases and 60 controls, and hence, applying the findings to the general population would be incorrect. Hence, it is always recommended to determine the confidence interval for the value of OR that we obtain. The confidence interval gives us a range into which likelihood of OR from other samples studied will be more and it then can indicate to the true population values. That becomes a practical and statistically sound approach.

For the finer details on OR you need to refer to your textbook on biostatistics. Here, we are primarily concerned with the giving conceptual clarity on OR in relation to case-control studies.

To get an idea of the practical implementation of this type of studies, one must refer to the case-control study on assessment of hazards of smoking, which was conducted in India. The study was nationwide, covered both women and men, and collected information on all adult deaths from 2001 to 2003 in a nationally representative sample of 1.1 million homes.[64]

Advantages of Case-Control Studies[45]

- Case-control studies can be done in lesser time and with lesser cost (in comparison to prospective cohort studies).
- With these type of studies, it is possible to investigate a wide range of suspected or probable risk factors.
- They are particularly suitable to investigate rare diseases or diseases with a long induction period.

Disadvantages of Case-Control Studies

- Selection of an appropriate control group becomes a problem many times, and this may allow selection bias to influence study findings.
- When we try to obtain the information on exposure in retrospect, it becomes difficult to ensure the accuracy of the information on past exposures (*information bias*).
- The temporal sequence between exposure and disease may be difficult to establish (*reverse causality*).
- These studies are not suitable for investigating rare exposures (unless the exposure is responsible for a large proportion of cases, i.e., the population excess fraction is high).
- It is not possible to obtain estimates of disease incidence among those exposed and those unexposed to a presumed risk factor (except if the study is general population-based).

COHORT STUDIES

A cohort is a group of individuals that have a common characteristics or exposure. We have seen in case-control studies that those who have already developed the effect or outcome (i.e., disease, for your reference) are usually traced backward, to understand exposure to a particular risk factor. In contrast to this, cohort studies are forward-looking or prospective studies.

In a cohort study, the epidemiologist records whether each study participant is exposed to a particular factor or not, and then follows the participants to see if they develop the disease in reference. The investigators or epidemiologists do not determine the exposure; they simply observe it to see the outcome. After a period, they compare the outcome (disease) in those who were exposed, with those who were not exposed.[5, 45]

In case-control studies, the selection of cases and controls depends on presence and absence of disease respectively, whereas in cohort studies those who are exposed are selected as cases, and those who are unexposed to the factor in reference are selected as controls. Disease occurrence rates in the group of unexposed persons enrolled in the study give us a baseline to make comparisons with that of the exposed persons enrolled. A significantly higher occurrence of disease in exposed persons shows that there is an association of the factor with the disease.

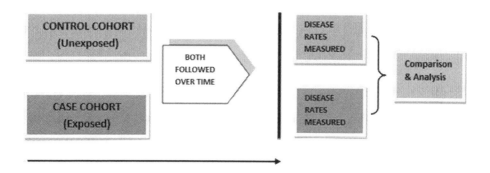

Figure 19: Scheme of a basic cohort study

As evident from the illustration in figure 19 above, follow-ups of cohort cases and controls are done in cohort studies. Hence these are also referred to as *follow up studies.* As these studies are carried out in a forward direction over a time period, hence also referred to as *prospective studies.*[1]

Cohort studies can be retrospective also, and such studies are known as *retrospective or historical cohort studies.*[1] The exposure has already occurred in the past, and the effect or outcome (disease) has also occurred.

We take a simple hypothetical example to understand it further. Suppose, we have a cement production industry from where 50 workers reported having manifestations like shortness of breath, wheezing and persistent cough. Complete Investigations of the persons revealed that 11 of them had Interstitial Lung Disease (ILD). Out of total fifty, besides the workers with ILD, 30 individuals had chronic bronchitis with acute exacerbation, and 9 had bronchial Asthma.

A retrospective cohort study was planned to understand what led to such high rates of respiratory manifestations in the workers' population. Matching Controls, who did not have a history of long exposure to pollutants of cement manufacturing unit, were selected. The clinical examination and investigations of controls revealed that five of them had chronic bronchitis, one had ILD, none had bronchial asthma. Both cohorts were traced forwards over a period beginning 15 years back to understand their history of exposures, illnesses, cigarette smoking habits, etc.

The findings revealed that consistent exposure to high levels of cement dust in cement manufacturing environment for periods more than 10 years was responsible for significantly higher rates of respiratory pathology, including ILD, among the industrial workers, suggesting a positive association. Please note, the example above is just a hypothetical example, modified using findings of a study on cement workers, given here to help you understand the concept.[65]

Analyzing Findings from Cohort Studies

For drawing inferences and understanding the risk that a particular factor contributes towards causation of a particular disease, we use following approaches;

1. Calculate and compare incidence rates of the disease or outcome in reference, for the group of exposed with that of unexposed persons.
2. Estimate risk of the outcome for group of exposed with that of unexposed persons.

Calculating incidence is done the way we have learned. Let us have a re-look to clarify it -

Table 7: Analyzing findings from cohort studies

Group	Disease Develops	Disease Does Not Develop	Total	Incidence
Exposed	a	b	a + b	$\frac{a}{a+b}$
Not exposed	c	d	C + d	$\frac{c}{c+d}$

Comparing incidence between *exposed* and *not exposed* will tell us whether the '*exposed*' group has a different incidence as compared to the '*not-exposed*' group. Based on these observations we can say that exposure to a particular factor was found to be associated with increased incidence of the disease under study.

Estimation of risk is done after we have arrived at the incidence rates for '*exposed*' and '*not exposed*' groups. We can do it by using the concepts of **Relative Risk** and **Attributable risk**.[1, 5]

Relative Risk (RR)

Although we have discussed Relative Risk (RR) concept in the section on Case-control studies, we will revisit it as it is of more relevance here. We are now putting some hypothetical values in table 8 and will use them to explain the concept. Before looking at the table, we should remember that Relative Risk is defined as the ratio of incidence among *exposed* to incidence among *non-exposed*.

Table 8: Calculating Relative Risk

Group	Disease Develops	Disease Does Not Develop	Total	Incidence	RR
Exposed	180 (a)	5304 (b)	5484 (a + b)	$\dfrac{180}{5484}$ = (0.0328)	$\dfrac{0.0328}{0.0109}$ = 3.0009
Not Exposed	21 (c)	1899 (d)	1920 (c + d)	$\dfrac{21}{1920}$ = (0.0109)	

A Relative Risk value of around 3 as obtained above, means that the exposed group has three times higher chances of developing the disease than the non-exposed group.[66] In other words, we can say that the exposed group has 200% higher chances of developing the disease in comparison to the non-exposed group.

There can be situations where the value of RR is equal to 1. This will happen when the numerator and the denominator, in the formula for calculating RR used above, are equal. That means the incidence of outcome/disease among 'exposed' and 'not-exposed' are equal. In other words, exposure to the particular factor in reference has no association with the disease under study.[66]

Let's now imagine a situation where RR value comes out to be less than 1. It will so happen in situations where the numerator, i.e., incidence among 'exposed' is less than the denominator, i.e., incidence among 'not-exposed.' We can call this a negative association.[45] It will be seen in circumstances where the factor under study has a protective role, for example, exposure to regular physical activity (e.g., brisk walking for 5 Kilometers everyday) and chances of cardiovascular diseases. We know that those who are exposed to the practice of regular physical activity will have comparatively lower chances of developing those cardio-vascular diseases which are lifestyle related (related to stress, sedentary life-lack of physical activity, diet, smoking, etc.).

Attributable Risk (AR)

This gives us the risk, of developing the disease under study, that can be attributed to the factor that is being investigated. Let's understand it through a simple example. Assume that in a study on lung cancer and smoking, we noted following observations as given in table 9;

Table 9: Understanding Attributable Risk

Group	Lung Cancer Develops	No Lung Cancer	Total	Incidence	RR
Exposed (Smokers)	7 (a)	93 (b)	100 (a + b)	$\frac{07}{100}$ = (0.07)	$=\frac{0.07}{0.01}$
Not Exposed (Non-Smokers)	1 (c)	99 (d)	100 (c + d)	$\frac{01}{100}$ = (0.01)	
A					= 7.00

Look at the highlighted column of 'incidence.' Had all the individuals in the exposed group been non-smokers, even in that situation one case of lung cancer for 100 individuals would have occurred in them, as we observe in the 'not-exposed' group. This means that additional 6 cases, which we are observing in the exposed group, can be attributed to smoking. So, the risk difference what we get here is the AR. Here is one more assumption, that all other factors have an equal role for both the groups in the causation.

Now, the next point is to know how is the AR calculated and expressed. The formula for calculating AR is as given below;

$$AR = \frac{\text{Incidence among exposed} - \text{incidence among not exposed}}{\text{Incidence among exposed}} \times 100$$

AR is expressed in terms of percentage.

Let's now put the values from our lung cancer example as mentioned in table 9 above;

$$AR = \frac{0.07 - 0.01}{0.07} \times 100 = 85.71\%$$

We have now got the value of AR. In the above example, AR is 85.71%. It's important to understand what does this value mean. This tells us that in our hypothetical study, 85.71 percent individuals had lung cancer due to their exposure to smoking. It is a strong cause-effect relationship. We can now very well imagine the importance that smoking carries if we want to address the problem of lung cancer effectively.

Some other terms that are commonly applied in reference to these studies are mentioned below;

Risk Difference;

The risk difference is the difference in rates of occurrence between exposed and unexposed groups in the population. This is a valuable mean to measure what is the extent of the public health problem caused by that particular exposure. This is also referred to as *excess risk*.

The Attributable Fraction (Exposed);

The attributable fraction (exposed), is the proportion of all cases that can be attributed to a particular exposure. If we divide the risk difference by incidence of outcome among exposed population, then we get the Attributable fraction (exposed). This is also known as the *etiological fraction (exposed)*. Attributable fractions are useful for assessing priorities for public health action whereas the AR is used on the study population. For example, we know that smoking and very high levels of air pollutants both can be responsible for lung pathologies like cancer of the lungs. After evaluating attributable fraction among exposed, separately for both these factors, if we come to know that the attributable fraction (exposed) is higher for smoking then we can set the priorities for public health action accordingly. Similarly, there can be multiple factors responsible for causing a disease which can be evaluated to understand the priorities.[5]

Population Attributable Risk;

The population-attributable risk (PAR) is the incidence of a disease in a population that is attributed to a given risk factor exposure. For example, we understand that health authorities know the incidence of lung cancer for the general population. We also know that it is a comprehensive measure of incidence among those who smoke and those who don't. Incidence among those who smoke would be higher in comparison to those who don't. General population incidence would be somewhere between these two extremes. Here, PAR can be calculated using the following formula-

$$PAR = \frac{\text{Incidence in total population - Incidence among unexposed}}{\text{Incidence in total population}}$$

PAR is useful for determining the relative impact that exposure has in producing the outcome for the total population. PAR tells us the proportions by which the incidence rate of the outcome (e.g., lung cancer) will be reduced in the total population, if we eliminate the exposure to the risk factor (e.g., smoking).[5]

Advantages of Cohort Studies

- Exposure is measured before disease onset and is therefore likely to be unbiased in terms of associated disease development.
- Rare exposures can be examined by appropriate selection of study cohorts.
- Multiple outcomes (diseases) can be studied for any one exposure.
- The incidence of the disease can be measured in the exposed and unexposed groups.[45]

Disadvantages of Cohort Studies

- They can be very expensive and time-consuming, particularly if conducted prospectively.

> Changes in exposure status and diagnostic criteria over time can influence the classification of individuals according to exposure and disease status.

> Ascertaining the outcome may be influenced by knowledge of the subject's exposure status (*information bias*).

> Losses to follow-up may introduce *selection bias*.[45]

This chapter is intended to give a conceptual clarity on approaches in analytical epidemiology. As students advance in their academic standards, it is recommended that they should practice developing some concept notes on various methods and try application of those in real-life studies in any discipline of their preference.

Points to Remember

- Design of case-control studies.
- Selection of cases, controls and matching.
- How is analysis of exposure disease association done.
- Odds Ratio.
- Merits & demerits of case-control studies.
- Cohort study design.
- Merits and demerits of cohort studies.
- Analysis of exposure disease association.
- Steps involved in calculation of Relative Risk and Attributable Risk.

CHAPTER
8

EXPERIMENTAL EPIDEMIOLOGY

Learning Objectives

- ❖ Understand broad approach and ojective of experimental epidemiological methods.
- ❖ Know what is randomized controlled trial (RCT).
- ❖ Examine the scheme of basic RCT and follow the logic.
- ❖ Know different tupes of RCT designes and understand the purpose of each of them.
- ❖ Learn what does blinding mean, what are different types.
- ❖ What are non randomized trials and what is their advantage?

We have seen in the observational/analytical studies that the epidemiologists observe and analyze the role a particular risk factor may have played in the causation of the disease under study. This is done in settings where there are already some people who are exposed to the risk factor, while there are others who are not exposed to it.

In experimental epidemiological studies, as the name suggests, there is some experimentation that is done. Experimentation means that the person doing the study is making some changes and trying to assess the impact of such changes on the outcome. These changes could be done with the risk factor exposure, individual behaviors, or interventions related to treatment or prevention. To understand the concept, we need to understand what kind of changes are done.

From our understanding of disease concepts in public health, we know that diseases have multifactorial causation. Controlling or changing individual risk factors and then analyzing the outcome can give us information about the extent to which the individual factors play a role in the causation of disease under study. For example, in the causation of heart diseases, cigarette smoking, lack of physical activity, diet all seem to play a role. Now assume that we take a group of people who are exposed to all these factors and tell some of the individuals to stop smoking, exercise regularly and follow the appropriate diet. Here we have deliberately made these changes. When we compare the outcome after a period, then we will come to know to what extent we were able to change the outcome in this subgroup by making changes in the exposure to risk factors.

Such experiments can be done in human subjects or animals. There are many ethical issues that influence the study protocols. For example, denying some treatment to a group of patients, for the sake of assessing its impact, becomes unethical. Similarly, knowingly and forcefully exposing people to something harmful just for the experimentation is unethical. So, the ethical component is one of the most important guiding principles of such experiments.

On the basis of designs of these studies and the way of experimenting, there can be following types of experimental studies-

1. Randomized controlled trials (RCTs)
2. Non-randomized trials

There are many sub-categories of each of these groups, specifically of RCTs, which we will discuss in subsequent sections.

RANDOMIZED CONTROLLED TRIALS (RCTs)

There are two important terms in this nomenclature, one, *'randomized'* and the other, *'controlled.'* The term *'Randomized'* indicates that the allocation of study subjects to intervention or control groups is randomly done and cannot be determined by the investigator. Suppose, in a school, there is a new teacher who claims that she uses improved and effective ways of teaching that have a positive impact on the performance of students. The head of the school wants this to be evaluated against the impact that existing teachers and their methodologies have on students' performance. If the investigator deliberately assigns all bright students to the new teacher's class, or to the existing other teacher's class, then it will create a huge bias. We can address this by randomly allocating students to the new and existing teachers in a manner that each student has an equal chance of getting allocated to any of these two classes. This is randomization, critically important for RCTs.[67, 68]

The term 'controlled' indicates that there is an arrangement of comparing the outcome in the intervention group with that of a matching control group. Also, it implies that there are predefined eligibility criteria, specified hypothesis to be tested, methods of enrollment and follow up, monitoring strategy and analysis plan.[69]

In brief, we can say that RCT is an epidemiological experiment which is designed to study the effect of a drug or treatment intervention or a preventive intervention on the health outcome.[5, 70]

Scheme of a Basic RCT

The illustration below (figure 20) shows a basic schematic representation of how a standard RCT looks. There can be many alterations in this basic arrangement which are carried out to give a new design to the RCT depending upon the objective with which any given study is to be carried out. We will come to know about this when we go through different categories of RCTs in subsequent sections. But, at this stage, it is important to understand the scheme of a basic RCT as given below;

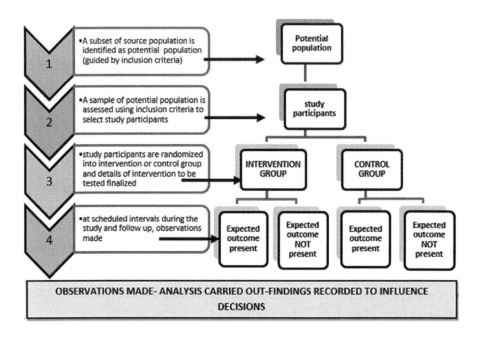

Figure 20: Basic scheme of a RCT

Types of RCTs

There are various factors on the basis of which we can classify RCTs. It is important for us to know at least the major types and the concepts. Classification can be based on following factors[71]-

1. Type of intervention that is to be evaluated.
2. Participants' exposure to the intervention.

3. Number of participants in the study.
4. Depending upon who knows what interventions are being administered when.

Based on each of these factors we will see which are the main subtypes in following sections.

Based on Type of Intervention That Is to Be Evaluated

I. Efficacy Vs. Effectiveness trials

Efficacy refers to whether an intervention works in the participants to whom it has been offered. The investigators want clear-cut evidence on this. At this stage of the investigation, they are not primarily interested to know how does a particular intervention work in those who are receiving it.

Effectiveness refers to how does a particular intervention work for those who have been offered it. These trials try to evaluate the effects of intervention in circumstances which clinicians encounter in their daily practice.[71]

II. Superiority Vs. Equivalence Trials

Very often, the trials are designed to evaluate whether one intervention, out of two interventions, is superior to the other. Such trials are known as superiority trials.[71]

Also, sometimes trials aim to ascertain whether a new intervention or drug is as effective as the existing one (equivalent). This is done if some alternative treatment regime is to be evaluated. These are known as equivalence trials.[71]

III. Phase I, Phase II or Phase III Trials

Phase I, II and III trials are meant for evaluating new drugs.

Phase I trials are the first series of trials that are conducted in human subjects in the course of evaluating a new drug. Human subjects are involved once the safety and efficacy of the drug are established on animals. These trials evaluate the safety of the drug in humans, determine the safe dosage range and also the side effects. Phase I trials are conducted on a small number of healthy volunteers (usually 20 to 80).[71, 72]

Phase II clinical trials are conducted after phase I trials are done. These trials are aimed at establishing the efficacy of different dose range and frequencies of administration of the drug under study. Although phase II trials are focused on the efficacy of a drug, these can provide additional information on its safety. If the drug under study turns out to be ineffective or it causes excess toxicity, then no more trials are conducted. Numbers of subjects engaged are usually in the range of a few hundred (100-300). These studies aren't large enough to show whether the drug will be beneficial. Instead, Phase II studies provide researchers with additional safety data. Researchers use these data to refine research questions, develop research methods, and design new Phase III research protocols.[71, 72]

Phase III trials, conducted once the efficacy and safety are established through phase II trials, are actually effectiveness trial. These evaluate the effectiveness of the new intervention or drug in comparison to the existing one. Also, Phase III studies provide most of the safety data. In previous studies, it is possible that less common side effects might have gone undetected. Because phase III studies are larger (300 to 3,000 participants) and longer in duration, the results are more likely to show long-term or rare side effects.[72]

The term 'phase IV trials' is also used sometimes. These trials are done to evaluate the side effects of a drug, once it has already been approved for marketing. Several thousand volunteers who have the disease/condition usually participate in phase IV trials.[72]

Based on Participants' Exposure to Intervention

I. Simple, Two Arm Parallel Trials

In parallel trials, one group of participants is exposed to the intervention to be evaluated (treatment/drug, etc.), and the other group, not exposed to that intervention, serves as a control. So, there are two separate parallel arms in the study.

Experimental Epidemiology

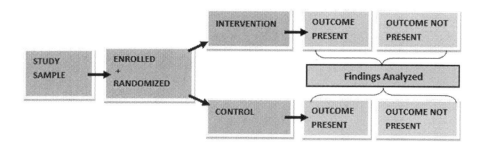

Figure 21: Simple two arm parallel trial

1. Crossover Trials

Suppose a new drug is to be evaluated to see whether this is effective in a stable chronic disease. Administration of this drug and observation of its effects is done in the intervention group. This needs to be compared with a control group, which receives only a placebo.[45]

Now, what is done in a cross-over trial is that for a certain period, the intervention group (intervention arm) will first receive the study drug and the control group will get a placebo (control arm). After a pre-decided observation period, study drug and placebo are stopped. A crossover RCT begins the same as a traditional RCT, however, after the end of the first treatment phase, each participant is re-allocated to the other treatment arm.[73] In a crossover approach, patients/subjects can act as their own controls, and at the same time, it is also possible to make comparisons between the two groups.[74]

It is important that, depending upon the pharmacological properties of the drug used, time is allowed to lapse so that there are no carryover effects of the drug in the intervention group. This is known as **wash-out period**.[74, 75] After the wash-out period, the control group, which was earlier receiving the placebo, will receive the study drug. Similarly, the intervention group, which was earlier receiving the study drug, will receive the placebo. Observation after this cross-over will be recorded again.

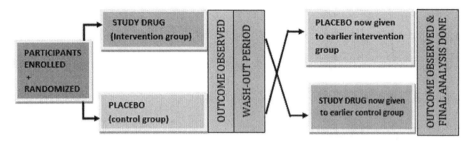

Figure 22: Cross-over trials

2. Factorial Trials

When two or more interventions or drugs are to be evaluated through comparison against each other and also with different controls, then Factorial RCT design is the answer.[45, 71]

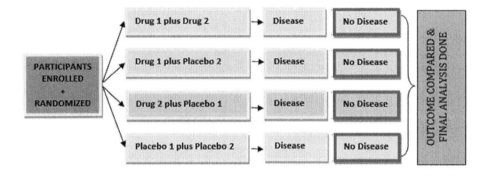

Figure 23: Factorial trial

From the illustration above we see that the findings can suggest whether drug 1 alone is better than the drug 2 or vice-versa. We will also know if the combination of drug 1 & drug 2 outperforms and is better than either drug 1 or drug 2 used alone.[76]

Based on Number of Participants in the Study

1. N-of-1 Trials

These can be single participant trials which follow the principle of cross-over trials in a sequential manner.[74] As we know in a cross-over trial a group gets one of the interventions or drugs to be studied and placebo in an alternating manner. Similarly, in N-of-1 trials, a subject gets the intervention or a drug for certain period, then it is withdrawn, and then other drug/intervention or placebo is started. We can do this with multiple drugs in a sequential manner and note the responses and decide which one produces the best results.[71, 77]

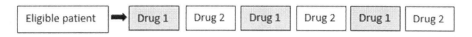

Figure 24: N-of-1 Trial

Above illustration (figure 24) denotes a situation where two drugs are being compared. The patient does not know which one is being administered when. Some placebo can also be introduced in between if it is so planned. There can be many repetitions until a final inference is reached. We can also tweak the doses and duration of each treatment if the further comparison between more than one duration or dose regimen is needed for the drugs under study.

2. Mega-Trials

As the name suggests, these are very large trials, often multi-centre, but the information to be collected is kept very simple. It is important to keep in mind the feasibility, cost and quality issues while designing such huge trials. Hence the data to be collected should be limited and uncomplicated.[78]

3. Sequential Trials

In these trials, the number of participants needed is not determined beforehand. These are studies with parallel designs, where one arm deals with one drug (or intervention) and the other arm with the other drug (or intervention) against which comparison is to be made, or this second arm could be a placebo (or control) arm. The subjects of the experimental group and the control group are arranged in pairs (one who receives the experimental treatment and the other who receives the reference treatment). After the interventions or drugs are administered, the subjects are assessed to evaluate the impact, and the findings are added to the results obtained up to that time.[79] Enrolment of subjects may continue until a conclusion is reached.

4. Who Knows What Interventions Are Being Administered

Depending on who all know which interventions/drugs are being administered during a trial and when are these being administered, we categorize trials into different categories. Let's have a look at different categories of people involved in any trial:

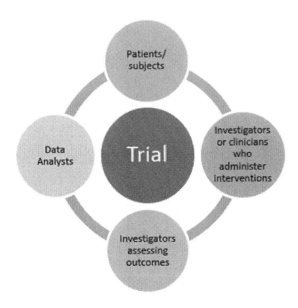

Figure 25: Key Stakeholders in a Clinical Trial

I. Open Trials

If all the stakeholders in a trial as shown in the illustration above (figure 25), are aware which intervention/drug is being administered at what time, such trials are known as Open trials. Sometimes, it is impossible to keep any of the stakeholders blind, as happens in case if a surgical intervention is being tried. Open trials have high chances of bias, as both the patient and the physician are aware of which groups are receiving what type of treatment.[80]

II. Single-Blind Trials

In this category of trials, either the participants or the investigators assessing the outcome are not knowing which intervention (or drug) is administered to whom and when.[81]

III. Double-Blind Trials

In double-blind trials, the participants, as well as the investigators assessing the outcome, are blinded, i.e., they do not know which intervention (or drug) is administered to whom and when.[81]

IV. Triple or Quadruple Blind Trials

If three or four of the groups, as shown in the illustration above (figure 25), are blinded then the trials are known as triple or quadruple blind trials.

Potential Benefits of Blinding

The process of blinding is helpful in eliminating biases at different levels. When the participants are blinded, chances of them having biased psychological or physical responses to the interventions (or drugs) are minimized. Also, they are more likely to comply with the trial regimens as they are not biased against one or other intervention (or drug) that is being tried.[82]

When the trial investigators are blinded, they are less likely to pass on their biases or experiences relating to a particular intervention (or drug) to the trial participants. Also, they are less likely to differentially adjust dose (if it's a drug trial). Such differential dose adjustment can happen if the investigators are not blinded, and this may influence the outcome.[67, 83]

When the outcome assessors are blinded, it becomes less likely that their own biases will impact the assessment of outcome. The highest possible degree of blinding should be chosen to minimize bias.[68]

NON-RANDOMIZED CONTROLLED TRIALS

Non-randomized controlled trials are those clinical trials where the study participants are not assigned to different groups through a random method. Either the participants themselves or the researchers can choose the group for each of the participants in a manner which is not random. In other words, it is a completely non-random allocation, hence the name.[84, 85]

These controlled trials are interventional study designs that compare a group where an intervention was performed with a group where there was no intervention. These are convenient study designs that are most often performed prospectively and can suggest possible relationships between the intervention and the outcome.[86]

We know from our section on RCTs that randomization reduces the chances of bias, as confounders can be controlled significantly. However, in non-randomized trials, since there is no randomization, the chances of bias are comparatively more.[83, 87]

Non-randomized trials come under the category of Quasi-experimental designs as they are not the true experimental designs.[83, 88] The question that arises is 'why do we then need non-randomized trials?'. It is primarily because of the reason that randomization may not be possible everywhere.[87] For example, in a surgical intervention, it is unethical to randomly assign a patient to an intervention which he or she does not want. From the ethical point of view, any surgeon planning to operate upon a patient will have to inform the procedure to the patient in details including possible risks and take his/her consent to operate. Also, it is impossible to keep the surgeon or patient blind (not aware which intervention is being carried out). In such situations, non-randomized trials become the choice. So, a non- randomized trial design is appropriate in the following broad conditions:[89]

> In situations where randomized allocation has a potential risk of reducing an intervention's effectiveness. This can happen when an intervention requires patient's active participation and compliance and this, in turn, will depend upon trust, belief and individual preference of the patient/study subject.

> When it would be unethical to do random allocation, as we discussed in the example of surgical intervention above or there are some legal restrictions.

> When cost or convenience factors make it impossible to do the random allocation.

In non-randomized controlled trials also, we need to go by proper selection criteria and study protocols, including inclusion and exclusion criteria, to ensure that the intervention and control groups are comparable to the extent that is practically possible. These criteria are generally not very restrictive. However, in non randomized trials also, there can be some medical, other scientific or ethical reasons on the basis of which we need to exclude subjects or patients.[90] As the selection criteria are generally not very stringent as in RCTs, it is possible with non-randomized trials to enroll a very large number of participants.

Generally, non-randomized trials have two groups, one is where intervention is being administered and the other without that particular intervention. The latter serves as the control group. For both the groups, we must obtain the baseline data on key variables. This data helps us verify the comparability of the two groups. Also, it helps us make comparisons relating to the impact of the intervention in reference. Such parallel controls enrolled for the study are known as *'concurrent controls.'* Concurrent controls are enrolled simultaneously with the treatment group from the same source population and followed for the same study period.[91]

There can also be non-randomized trials with no control arm, i.e., a single arm non-randomized trial. But it does not mean that we are not in a position to make comparisons. In such situations, the comparisons are made using *'historical controls.'* For example, if some improved drug or intervention is to be tried, its impact is measured against that of an existing drug or intervention which was used in a comparable set of patients with the same disease at some point of time in the past. Historical control is a subject treated at some time in past, with the standard form of care, against which the treatment under investigation is to be compared.[91]

We know that for RCTs the selected trial site should have a high ability to conduct such trials. But, in case of non-randomized trials using clearly defined study protocols, we can enroll as many sites as required to achieve the required sample size. We can enroll multiple hospitals, health centers or practitioners. In that way, the results of such trials become more relevant for a wider population. However, non-randomized trials cannot test exposure-outcome (cause and effect) hypothesis; they can be used for showing disease trends and associations.[88]

There are two key parameters which should always be borne in mind while designing and conducting a non-randomized controlled trial. These are; (i) generalizability or external validity and (ii) internal validity. These criteria are relevant for Randomized Controlled Trials also but are being discussed here as these often become questionable in reference to Non-Randomized Controlled Trials.

Generalizability or external validity indicates the degree to which the selected sample is representative of the reference population or the population group to which the results of the trial would be applied. In other words, we can say this indicates the degree to which the study results hold true (can be applied) in other settings,[83] i.e., outside the study sample. That is why it is important to pay attention to the process of sample selection in such trials. If a sample is truly representative of given population, then the findings of such sample based trial would apply to the population it represents. Sometimes, the investigators tend to overlook this aspect for their convenience, and that adversely affects the generalizability of study findings.[88]

Internal validity refers to the degree to which the findings of the study represent the impact of the intervention, rather than the effect of external factors that can confound the results. In other words, it indicates the degree of reliability with which the results of intervention under study can be regarded as truly attributable to that intervention.[83, 87] Therefore, it is important to control the confounding factors to the maximum possible level. Two key areas should be kept in mind for improving the internal validity of a trial, first is *allocation bias* and the other is *preference*.

In RCTs, effects of allocation bias and preference can be significantly neutralized through proper randomization. But in non-randomized trials, care should be taken to control adverse effects of these two factors on trial findings.[88] Allocation bias creeps in when the subjects/participants allocated to receive the intervention under study are different in characteristics from those who are allocated to the control group (those receiving standard or existing intervention or not receiving any intervention).[87] Similarly, preferential allocation of a subject by the investigator, to a particular group for any reason, or subject's preference to be in a particular group for some reason, may disturb the comparability of the intervention group with the control group and the bias creeps in.

We know it is impossible to use RCTs in every situation. Hence, non-randomized trials offer a very good alternative in such scenarios. What is important while using non-randomized studies is to adhere to sample selection, group allocation, control of confounders, analysis and reporting guidelines if we want to have a high degree of reliability on the findings of these trials. We must remember that non-randomized trials are not a short-cut route to evaluate interventions.

 Points to Remember

- Concept of Randomized controlled trials.
- Basic scheme of RCT.
- Classification schemes of RCTs and different types.
- Phase- I, II, III and IV trials.
- Types of blinding.
- Benefits of blinding.
- Open trials.
- Simple two arms trials.
- Factorial trials.
- Crossover trials.
- N-of-1 trials.
- Mega trials.
- Sequential trials.
- Non-randomized controlled trials and their advantages.

CHAPTER

9

CAUSATION IN EPIDEMIOLOGY

Learning Objectives

- Understand the concept of causation analysis in epidemiology.
- Know about the stregth of causation.
- Learn about different factors in causation.
- Understand the criteria for establishing causal relation.
- Get basic idea about suitability of different epidemiological methods to prove causation.

In epidemiology, analyzing causes of diseases, injuries or other health conditions is important. Sometimes we analyze different factors and study what all effects exposure to those factors can have on the individuals. At many times, we start with persons already affected by a disease or a health condition and then try to find out what could have caused it. In either case, the intention is to gather the information which guides us in developing new prevention and control strategies to protect people, and improved treatment interventions to improve the overall outcome for those who are affected by a particular disease.

In public health, we understand that the diseases are caused by the interaction of multiple factors, which we call as 'multifactorial causation.' Some causes may play a stronger role than the others. The ultimate goal is to identify such causes and develop solutions to modify exposure to them so that the outcomes can be favorably changed. However, for establishing causation certain criteria are used as tools. These are discussed in the following paragraphs.

STRENGTH OF CAUSAL FACTORS

We define the cause of a disease, health condition or injury as a condition or event or characteristic or a combination of these factors, which produces the outcome (i.e., disease, health condition or injury). Characteristically, the cause must precede the outcome. Such causes can be put into different categories. A cause is considered as *sufficient* if it inevitably produces the outcome. This can be a gradual or abrupt process. When we say that a particular cause is *necessary*, then it means that the outcome cannot be produced when this cause is absent.[5, 92]

When we say that a particular cause is sufficient in the causation of some disease, it does not mean that cause is the sole factor. There can be multiple factors integrated into that single cause which are interdependent.[5] If a cause is identified, then, to begin with, it is not necessary, or it may not be practically possible to identify every factor integrated into that cause. Identification of the cause in totality is also helpful if removal of that cause reduces the disease burden. Further research will help us identify more and more individual factors that are integrated into that single cause.

FACTORS IN CAUSATION

It is important to understand different categories of factors that play specific roles in disease causation. These factors can be predisposing factors, enabling or disabling factors, precipitating factors and reinforcing factors.[5, 93] These categories are discussed in brief in the section below;

Predisposing Factors:

These are the factors which create a state of susceptibility, making the individual vulnerable to the get affected by a certain condition. For example, poor socio-economic condition predisposes children to get malnourished. Age, sex, race, genetic makeup, etc. are some other common examples that may result in certain conditions which make individuals prone to developing a particular disease or health condition.[5]

Enabling Factors:

Enabling factors are those factors that help an individual or family or society to adopt positive approaches for improving their health. For example, information on diet control and self-care is an enabling factor for people with diabetes which will help them lead a healthy life.

Precipitating Factors:

These the factors or conditions that trigger the onset of a certain health or medical condition or disease. For example, in hypersensitive individuals use of certain perfume sprays can precipitate asthma.

Reinforcing Factors:

These are the factors which either in a positive or in a negative way have an add-on effect on enabling or predisposing factors. For example, for an obese individual, having information on diet and exercise regimen can be an enabling factor whereas strong family and peer group support becomes a reinforcing factor.

It is interesting to note that, many times when more than one factors are involved in the causation of a disease, then the effect of these factors acting together is much more than the sum of the effect of individual factors. This is known as interaction among the causes.

ESTABLISHING A CAUSAL RELATION

If a factor is found to be associated with some disease, it is considered simply an association, unless it is proved to be a causal relation. To establish a causal relation, meticulous consideration of some essential criteria is required. Sir Austin Bradford Hill proposed following set of criteria, also known as Hill's criteria;

Temporal Association:

Temporal in this reference means something that is in accordance with time (time-related). With temporal association, we mean that any cause and its effect are as per time-related order, i.e., the cause always appears first and is followed by its effect.[94, 95, 96]

Plausibility:

Word plausible means something that is probable, reasonable or imaginable. A plausible association refers to an association which is consistent with other available scientific knowledge. For example, assume that a drug was shown to produce liver changes in an experimental animal in scientific laboratory experiments. This knowledge gives us reason to believe that it may be causing the same effect in human subjects who are receiving that drug. In many situations, like in new emerging diseases, there is no prior knowledge available to corroborate. Initially, the association may appear implausible because of non-availability of scientific information, but may eventually become plausible as relevant scientific information is gathered through experiments.[5, 94, 96]

Consistency:

If several studies or experiments conducted on the associated factor and its outcome, under different conditions, produce the same effect then we can say that there is consistency in the cause and effect. But, it is important to remember that wide variations in the levels of exposure to the factor under study, or some other factors that are peculiar to a particular host, may produce outcomes that appear inconsistent. In such scenario, a causal relation cannot be ruled out. This requires further experiments and analysis.[94, 96, 97]

Strength of Association:

A cause and effect relationship which shows a high relative risk is considered to be strong. A relative risk 2 or more indicates this. In a weak association, it is unlikely that there is a causal relationship between the exposure and outcome. In such relation, the incidence among exposed may appear to be more than that in non-exposed probably because of some bias or because of some confounding factors that could not be controlled.[5, 95]

Dose-Response Relationship:

If a study is conducted in an unbiased manner and we observe that reduced exposure to the suspected cause under study reduces the occurrence of the outcome. Under this situation, we can say that there is a dose-response relationship. Also, increase in the occurrence of the outcome upon increasing exposure to the suspected factor reflects a dose-response relationship.[5, 95]

Reversibility:

Removal of suspected cause reduces the occurrence of an outcome, this is known as reversibility. Suppose, an individual develops asthmatic bronchitis-like symptoms when exposed to tobacco smoke and removal of this exposure reduces the occurrence of these symptoms, then this is reversibility.[94, 98]

PROVING CAUSATION

After having acquainted ourselves with different types of epidemiological methods and having understood the concept of causation, we must also know which method is most suitable for proving any causal link.

Randomized controlled trials have a strong ability to prove causation. These trials can be suitably designed to verify most attributes of causation as discussed above.

The first indication or evidence towards the possibility of causation generally comes from observational studies, which can be further confirmed by experimental studies, i.e., randomized controlled trials.

Through proper study design, if we control biases then the case-control studies can also be used for proving causation. These studies may be preferred next to the randomized controlled trials. But, comparatively, their strength is considered moderate for this purpose.

Cross-sectional studies have limited ability to prove causation. In case of some constraints, if information from cross-sectional studies is to be utilized for proving causation, then care should be taken to understand exposure to the factor under study. The timing of exposure in reference to the timing of outcome is also important.

 Points to Remember

- Difference between a Sufficient cause and a necessary cause.
- Different type of factors that operate in causation.
- Different Criteria that are used for establishing a causal relationship.
- Ability of different epidemiological methods to prove causation.

CHAPTER
10

SCREENING FOR DISEASE

Learning Objectives

- ❖ Get conceptual clarity about screening for diseases.
- ❖ Know what different screening approaches are.
- ❖ Understand the key requirements for planning and implementation of screening.
- ❖ Understand how the accuracy of a screening test is determined.
- ❖ Learn the concept of sensitivity, specificity, positive and negative predictive value in reference to screening.

You must have experienced that when we try to enter a high-security establishment, the security officials check every individual to see if he or she is carrying any dangerous article along (like arms or ammunition, explosive material, corrosive liquids, dangerous drugs, etc.). Such material can be potentially used to inflict harm on others. You must have also observed that every person entering that establishment is checked, irrespective of whether that person has some criminal record in the past or not. This process is known as *'frisking'* and is a common site at the airports, Parliament house, defense establishments and at many places of importance. The purpose here is to find out potentially harmful individuals out of apparently harmless individuals.

Screening for diseases is also somewhat similar approach. Public health authorities want diseases to be detected early, treat them promptly and take adequate measures to prevent the spread of these diseases to other susceptible individuals. In case of non-communicable diseases, the idea is to eliminate or control the risk factors and treat the diseases early before they cause extensive irreversible harm to the affected individuals.

Coming back to the example of frisking mentioned above, you must have noticed that many times, security person use different measures- you are asked to pass through a door frame metal detector, then frisked manually and also using a hand-held metal detector. Similarly, if the need arises, we can use multiple methods for screening also. We will see what does that mean, in relevant sections of this chapter.

Before we arrive at the specific discussion on screening, there is another example which is worth considering here. Suppose, police persons catch hold of somebody from a gang of dacoits. When the person is frisked, there is a likelihood of finding ammunition/firearms/explosives/knife or any such material. But when the general public is frisked, everyone is looked at with suspicion, but only a few may be found carrying such dangerous items. Somewhat similar is the scenario for screening for diseases. We will understand its resemblance with screening in the following sections.

SCREENING

Screening is a highly valuable tool that helps us detect diseases early and treat them promptly. The commission on Chronic Illness (CCI) defines screening as "presumptive identification of an unrecognized disease or defect by rapidly applying certain tests, examinations, or other procedures." Screening tests separate out apparently well persons who probably have an unrecognized disease from those who do not have it. A screening test is not intended to be a diagnostic test. Persons with positive or suspicious findings on the application of screening test must be referred to their physicians for diagnosis and necessary treatment.[99, 100]

We have to understand that the screening tests are applied on asymptomatic or apparently healthy individuals. Therefore, these tests can detect the pre-clinical or subclinical phase of disease or early clinical phase where the individual screened could not notice the early manifestations. Contrary to these, the diagnostic tests are applied to individuals who are reporting to a clinician with complaints and some manifestations of a disease.

As we know, there are wide variations in the natural history of one disease from that of another. How a disease affects people, for how long it remains inapparent, how much time it takes to manifest, when does it reach a stage where irreversible damage is caused, or treatment becomes ineffective, etc. are the points that play an important role in deciding any screening strategy.

The illustration below (figure 26 and 27) will help us understand the dynamics of screening with some more clarity:

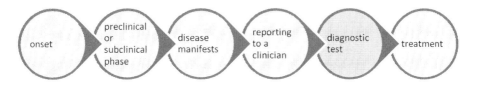

Figure 26: Usual time lapsed in getting a disease diagnosed

We know that in the above scenario, the affected individual gets the relevant diagnostic test done only when the clinicians advice so. In the above illustration, dark grey colored circle denotes the time when the diagnosis is made in clinical settings. Now, the question that arises in our minds is; can't we detect the disease much earlier than that? The answer is, yes!

We already know the key benefits of early detection of diseases. First, if it is an infectious disease, then detecting early will help us take measures to stop its spread to other persons, through appropriate prevention and control strategies. Secondly, in the communicable as well as in non-communicable diseases, we want to minimize the harm caused by the diseases among those affected and therefore want to treat it early. Those individuals who get complete and effective treatment in a prompt manner, can recover and can come back to their healthy state. We don't want the disease to reach a stage when it has already caused too much damage, and the treatment will no longer be effective. This stage is known as the **critical point**. There can be other critical points before this, which signify different stages of a disease.

As we know, diseases often become detectable much before they manifest clinically. There can be many biomarkers indicating towards disease, that can be detected as early as the inapparent phase (preclinical/subclinical phase) using some simple tests. If we screen individuals early, (during inapparent phase) provided disease has become detectable, we will get an indication that a particular person is developing the disease. Such tests are used as screening tests. Let's now look at the illustration below;

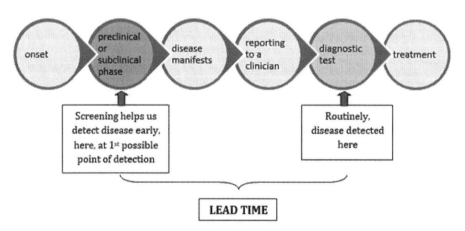

Figure 27: Screening test and its benefit

As depicted in the illustration above (figure 27), the time gained, or time advanced in detecting the disease early through screening, from its usual detection time through a diagnostic test which is done after the disease manifests, is known is the **Lead time.**

Having understood the basics, we will now go into some other details of screening in subsequent sections.

Types of Screening

There are different types of screening approaches which are used on the basis of requirements of a given situation. We have given subtle indication to these types in our example on 'frisking' in initial few paragraphs of this chapter.[5, 99, 100]

I. Mass Screening:

This indicates a screening strategy where either the entire population in reference or a group of it, is screened. No specific selection of any of the segments or subgroups of the population that is done under this approach.

II. Selective or Targeted Screening:

Some people or groups of people are at higher risk of developing particular diseases. Examples include clients of commercial sex workers for sexually transmitted diseases, injectable drug users for blood-borne infections, people working in cement/asbestos industry for obstructive airway diseases, etc. Strategy for screening such high-risk groups for concerned diseases is known as selective or targeted screening.

III. Multiple or Multiphasic Screening:

There is an example in initial page of this chapter, of security persons using multiple devices for frisking individuals. Somewhat similar approach is used in multiphasic screening. It is defined as the application of two or more screening tests, in combination, to a population group.[101, 102]

IV. Opportunistic Screening or Case Finding:

When patients visit a hospital for consulting a doctor for some disease or health condition and at that time they are screened for something other than the reason for which they primarily visited, is known as opportunistic screening.

Besides this, there can be various other ways of case finding, like surveillance, population-based surveys or specific screening of hospital patients. We will discuss these at appropriate places in the relevant sections.

Key Requirements for Planning and Implementing Screening

The foremost point for consideration while planning and developing a screening program for any disease is that the disease under consideration, if not detected early, will cause significant damage to the affected individual, to the community and also to the public health system. Besides this pivotal point, there are some other criteria which should be considered. These criteria are summarized in table 10 below;

Table 10: Screening-related criteria

Criteria Related to the Disease or Medical Condition	
Disease or medical condition	Very well defined from public health and clinical point of view
Existing burden of that disease or medical condition in the community	Some idea of the burden should be there, at least in terms of prevalence or incidence
Natural history of the disease	It is an important disease or condition from public health point, effective treatment or another remedy available. Also, basic epidemiological characteristics of the disease are known

Screening for Disease

Criteria Related to the Screening Test (Operational Part)	
Choice of the test	The tests should be simple and easy to administer
Test administration	Those carrying out the test are properly trained, specifically on the quality control aspect of it
Test values	Range or test results to differentiate affected and not affected are known
Cost of test	Screening would require large number of tests to be performed. Hence the test must be economical/cost effective
Acceptability	The test should be acceptable to those being screened and also to those who administer it
Post-test plan	What is to be done when a person tests positive should be defined and known to all concerned
Criteria for the Screening Test Itself (Technical & Quality Related)	
Reliability	The test should be so that it provides consistent results
Validity	The test should be able to correctly differentiate people into groups of those with disease and those without the disease.
Accuracy-Accuracy of a test is ascertained by;	Test should be able to produce accurate results
Sensitivity Specificity	These two qualities are discussed in details below

Accuracy of Screening Tests

The accuracy of a screening test is described in terms of sensitivity and specificity.[103] To understand the concepts of sensitivity and specificity, we will take some hypothetical examples and consider four different scenarios;

Our hypothetical example here is that out of 20 people in a village; there are 05 people who got a particular disease, remaining 15 are free from that disease.

Scenario 1:

All twenty people are screened using a highly accurate screening test. The test results came out positive for 05 persons and negative for remaining others, i.e., for 15. The numbers exactly match the figures in our example, which is a reference scenario for us. This is an ideal scenario where the screening test is correctly showing all positives as positives and all negatives as negatives. There is no erroneous or false result.

Refer to the illustration (figure 28) below. All solid black circles represent negative test results of the screening test applied; the solid black triangles represent positive test results.

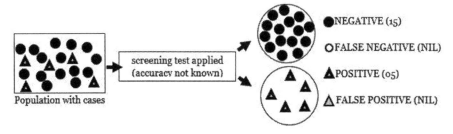

Figure 28: Screening outcome-scenario 1

Scenario 2:

Now, look at the illustration (figure 29) below. The picture here is somewhat different from that in scenario 1. The group to be screened has 5 positives and 15 negatives as in scenario 1. These are the actual numbers of positives and negatives. Here, the screening test applied was of lesser accuracy. The outcome of the test shows that there are 17 persons reported as negatives (free from disease) and 03 persons as positives (having the disease), against the actual numbers 15 and 05 respectively.

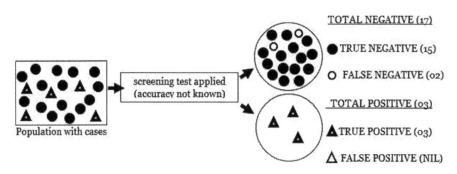

Figure 29: Screening outcome-scenario 2

So, we can say that there are no false positives here, but two of the positives are reported as negatives, i.e., 2 are false negatives. Now we should understand two important terms related to test accuracy and try to apply that concept in our example. The terms are **'Sensitivity'** and **'specificity'** which are explained below;

Sensitivity:

In reference to screening or diagnostic tests, sensitivity means the ability of a test to identify those who have a given disease. If 100 persons with the disease are tested, then, in order be categorized as '100% sensitive', the test used should detect all one hundred persons as positives.[5, 99, 104]

In our example from illustration (Figure 29) above, we are assuming that in a group of 20 people, only 5 have the given disease and rest 15 are free from that disease. Out of 5 who are actually positive, the test could show only 3 positives, and in place of 15 who are actually negative, it shows 17 as negatives (15 -true negatives,02 false negatives). There is no negative which is shown as positive. So, summarily, the results are;

True Positives=03   *False Positives=NIL*
True Negatives=15   **False Negatives=02**

We calculate sensitivity as below;

$$Sensitivity = \frac{True\ Positives}{(True\ Positives + False\ Negatives)} \times 100\ (result\ expressed\ as\ percentage)$$

Putting the values from our example,

$$Sensitivity = \frac{03}{(03 + 02)} \times 100 = \mathbf{60\%}$$

We can say that, with decreasing ability of a test to correctly show actual positives as positive test results, its sensitivity reduces.

Specificity:

With specificity, we mean a test's ability to correctly identify those who **do not** have a given disease. In other words, the test should give negative results for those who do not have the disease for which the test is being done.[5, 99, 104]

From our example from illustration (Figure 29) above, we know the following results;

True Positives=03   **False Positives=NIL**
True Negatives=15   False Negatives=02

The formula for calculating specificity of a test is as below;

$$Specificity = \frac{True\ Negatives}{(True\ Negatives\ +\ False\ Positives)} \times 100\ (result\ expressed\ as\ percentage)$$

Now, we put the values from our example into this formula;

$$Specificity = \frac{15}{(15\ +\ 00)} \times 100 = \mathbf{100\%}$$

From this derivation, we can conclude that a test that does not give any false positive result is 100% specific. In other words, if a test correctly identifies those free from disease as negatives only, then it is highly specific.

Scenario 3:

Look at the following illustration (Figure 30). Here again, we are using the assumption which we used in the example in scenario 1, i.e., there is a group of 20 persons, having 5 individuals who have the given disease and remaining 15 are free from it. But, the test outcomes are different in this scenario. Please refer to the numbers for different category of test outcomes mentioned in the illustration below;

Screening for Disease

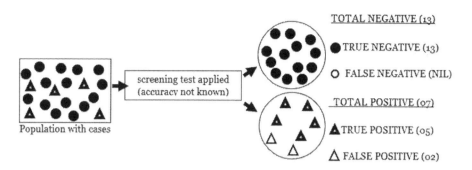

Figure 30: Screening outcome- scenario 3

The summary of results in Scenario 3 (figure 30) example is as below;

True Positives=05   *False Positives=02*
True Negatives=13   **False Negatives=NIL**

Let's calculate **sensitivity** of the test for this scenario;

$$Sensitivity = \frac{True\ Positives}{(True\ Positives + False\ Negatives)} \times 100\ (result\ expressed\ as\ percentage)$$

$$Sensitivity = \frac{05}{(05+00)} \times 100 = \mathbf{100\%}$$

Compare the result with scenario 1 sensitivity.

Based on this result, we can say that a test which does not show even a single person having a disease as negative, is highly sensitive. In other words, a test with no false negative result is 100% sensitive.

Now, we will calculate **Specificity** for scenario 3;

True Positives=05   **False Positives=02**
True Negatives=13   *False Negatives=NIL*

$$Specificity = \frac{True\ Negatives}{(True\ Negatives + False\ positives)} \times 100\ (result\ expressed\ as\ percentage)$$

$$\text{Specificity (Scenario 2)} = \frac{13}{(13 + 02)} \times 100 = \mathbf{86.66\%}$$

Here we can say that a test with increasing number of false positive results becomes less specific.

Scenario 4:

This scenario is a combination of scenario 2 and scenario 3. Please refer to the illustration below (Figure 31);

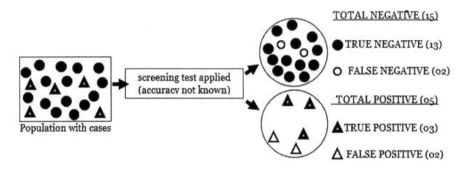

Figure 31: Screening outcome-scenario 4

Summary of the results in scenario 4:

True Positives=03   False Positives=02
True Negatives=13   **False Negatives=02**

$$\text{Sensitivity} = \frac{03}{(03 + 02)} \times 100 = \mathbf{60\%}$$

True Positives=03   **False Positives=02**
True Negatives=13   False Negatives=02

$$\text{Specificity} = \frac{13}{(13 + 02)} \times 100 = \mathbf{86.66\%}$$

Hopefully, you are now clear about the concept of sensitivity and specificity. What we need to remember is that in the ideal scenario, anyone would like to choose a test that is 100% sensitive and 100% specific. However, in a practical scenario, this becomes difficult. We will have to make some compromise either for sensitivity or specificity, depending on our requirements. For example, if we don't want to miss even a single person having a disease then some highly sensitive test should be chosen. Similarly, if we want that no person without disease should be shown as false positive, then we should select a highly specific test.

There are few more concepts related to screening tests. Two of them are worth discussing here.

Positive predictive value (PPV)

By definition, the positive predictive value of a test is the percentage of true positive results, out of all positives that it yields. So, the numerator is true positive results, and the denominator is the sum of true positive and false positive results.[5, 100, 105] However, these are the numbers obtained through predictions using experimental results of the test to understand sensitivity and specificity, and not after we know the results from actual screening activity. The formula would be;

$$Positive\ predictive\ value = \frac{True\ Positives}{(True\ Positives\ +\ False\ Positives)}$$

Now, the question that arises in our minds is how to arrive at these predictions. Let's take an example to understand this. We assume that we are using a test that has 95% sensitivity and 95% specificity. A test of 95% sensitivity would help us detect 95% of positive results as true positives, remaining 5% could be false negatives. Whereas, with 95% specificity we mean that the test would report 95% of all negatives as true negatives and remaining 5% could be false positives.

Let's take another assumption about a disease to be screened, which has a low prevalence, say, 1%. For this disease, out of 100 individuals screened, there is a likelihood that we will find 1 positive case.

With a test of 95% sensitivity (95/100), out of 1 positive case, the likelihood of getting true positive result will be;

= 1 X 0.95 = **0.95**

With a 95% specific test, out of total negatives (i.e., 100-1=99), number of false positives that may arise would be;

= 99 X (5/100) = 99 X 0.05 = **4.95**

Now, applying the formula, we will get the following;

= 0.95/(0.95 + 4.95)
= 0.16

For expressing it as percentage, we will multiply by 100,

= 0.16 X 100 = **16%**

This means that the positive predictive value of a test with 95% sensitivity and 95% specificity when used for screening a disease that has 1% prevalence, would be 16%

To understand the relation of the positive predictive value of a test with the prevalence of the disease which is to be screened, we will take another example. Let's assume that we want to use the same test (95% sensitivity and 95% specificity) in a situation where the prevalence of the disease is high, let's say, 10%;

With a test of 95% sensitivity (95/100), out of 10 positive cases, the likelihood of getting true positive result will be;

= 10 X 0.95 = **9.5**

With a 95% specific test, out of total negatives (i.e., 100-10=90), number of false positives that may arise would be;

= 90 X (5/100) = 90 X 0.05 = **4.5**

Now, the positive predictive value in this situation would be;

= 9.5/(9.5 + 4.5)
= 0.6785

Expressing it in percentage would make it;

= 0.6785 X 100 = **67.85**

The same test, when applied to a low prevalence situation shows lower Positive Predictive Value.

Negative Predictive Value (NPV)

Negative predictive value is also a predictive value, and it tells us about the likely proportion of true negative results out of the total negative results. The *numerator* is true negative results, and the *denominator* is the sum of true negative and false negative results. In simpler words, it reflects the probability of a person not having the disease, when the test result is negative.[5, 104, 105] The formula would be;

$$\text{Negative predictive value} = \frac{\text{True Negatives}}{(\text{True Negatives} + \text{False Negatives})}$$

Here also, to understand the calculations, we assume that we are using a test which has 95% sensitivity and 95% specificity, and the disease prevalence is 1%.

From the sensitivity percentage of 95, we know that the test can give true positive results for 95% of those with disease Remainder 5% maybe reported as negatives which are 'false negatives.' Similarly, from 95% specificity, we understand that for 95% of people without the disease, the test will give true negative results, and for remaining 5% without disease, it may give false positive results. Since the prevalence is assumed to be 1%, we would get 10 positive cases out of 1000. Let's put this stepwise;

Total population screened: 1000
Likely positive cases: 10
Likely negative cases; 990 (1000-10)

Now, we will try to predict false negative (those who are positive, but result shows them as negatives) cases;

False negatives are likely to be around 5% of all positives;

False negatives = 10 X (5/100)
= 0.5

Since the test is 95% specific, likelihood of getting true negatives out of all negatives would be

$$= 990 \ X \ (95/100)$$
$$= 940.5$$

$$Negative \ predictive \ value = \frac{True \ Negatives}{(True \ Negatives + False \ Negatives)}$$

$$= 0.9994$$

This value is required to be expressed as percentage;

$$= 0.9994 \ X \ 100$$
$$= \mathbf{99.94\%}$$

We will now take an example of a comparative higher prevalence i.e. 10% and calculate Negative Predictive Value;

Total population screened: 1000
Likely positive cases: 100 (at prevalence 10%)
Likely negative cases; 900 (1000-100)

False negatives are likely to be around 5% of all positives;

False negatives = 100 X (5/100)
= 5

Since the test is 95% specific, likelihood of getting true negatives out of all negatives would be

$$= 900 \times (95/100)$$
$$= 855$$

$$\text{Negative predictive value} = \frac{\text{True Negatives}}{(\text{True Negatives + False Negatives})}$$

$$\text{Negative predictive value} = \frac{855}{(855 + 5)}$$

$$= 0.9942$$

This value should be expressed as percentage;

$$= 0.9942 \times 100$$
$$= \mathbf{99.42\%}$$

Therefore, we can say that for a given sensitivity and specificity, the **negative predictive value of a test decreases with increase in prevalence** *and its* **positive predictive increases with increase in prevalence.**

Here is a graphical illustration which tries to show this relation. This illustration was made using an example of 1000 person with different levels of prevalence of a disease (6%, 10%, 20% and 30%). It was assumed that the sensitivity and specificity both were at 80% (which is not a practical scenario). This is being shown here just to give a visual impression of the inter-relation of prevalence with PPV and NPV;

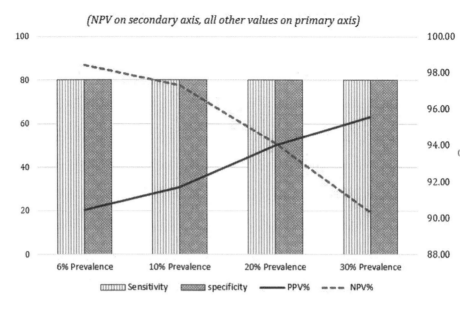

Figure 32: Hypothetical Example Showing Effect of Prevalence on PPV and NPV

For a given prevalence, when the sensitivity of test increases then the percentage of true positives would be more and this will increase its PPV. A graphical presentation of a hypothetical example in the illustration below (figure 33) would give us a visual impression;

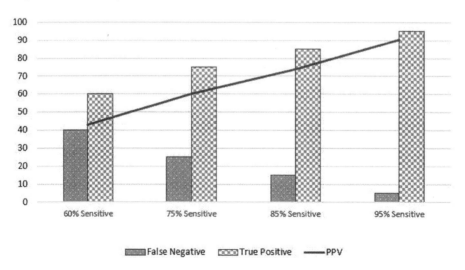

Figure 33: Hypothetical Example Showing Effect of Sensitivity on Positive Predictive Value

When the specificity of test increases (and the prevalence is assumed to be constant) then it will give more true negatives and this will result into an increase of its NPV. The relation is shown through a hypothetical example in figure 34 below;

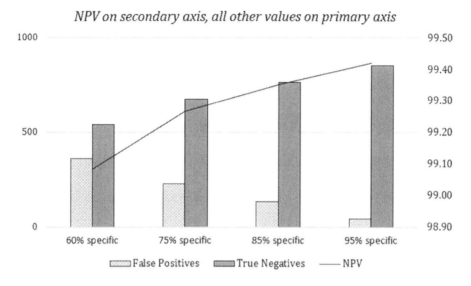

Figure 34: Hypothetical Example Showing Effect of Specificity on Negative Predictive Value

What we need remember here is that the above examples and graphical illustrations have tried to explain sensitivity and PPV, specificity and NPV separately. But in actual scenario we need to consider sensitivity and specificity together to decide for selecting a given test for screening. The above explanations were separately illustrated for explaining the relations with prevalence and predictive values.

From the following illustration (figure 35) we will get an idea about inter-relation of these values.

We can note that false positive rates affect specificity as well as PPV. Similarly, false negative rates have a bearing on NPV and sensitivity as well. All these factors help us decide which test to choose in what situation.

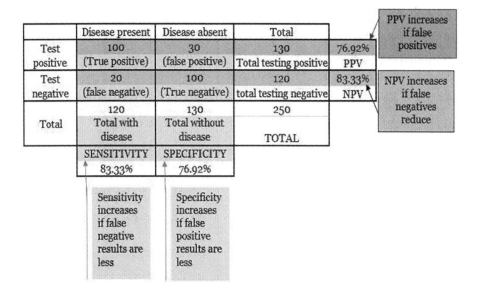

Figure 35: Interplay of sensitivity, specificity, PPV and NPV

 Points to Remember

❖ Concept of screening for disease.

❖ Different types of screening.

❖ Key requirements for planning and implementation of screening for disease:

- Medical condition related criteria.
- Screening test related criteria (operational part).
- Technical and quality criteria related to screening test.

❖ Accuracy of screening test and related measures.

- Sensitivity.
- Specificity.
- Positive predictive value.
- Negative predictive value.

CHAPTER

11

INVESTIGATING AN EPIDEMIC

Learning Objectives

- ❖ Understand different factors which are useful for epidemiologists in deciding about investigating an epidemic.
- ❖ Know different steps that we should follow for investigating an epidemic.

We already know that outbreaks, clustering or epidemics of diseases are abnormal events. We utilize the usually existing frequency of any disease, to make comparisons and decide if there is any sudden increase in the number of cases of the given disease, or if there is any alarming change in its distribution pattern.

The occurrence of epidemics is a public health emergency and needs to be addressed immediately to prevent and control morbidity and mortality in the affected population. In order to understand the causes or factors that lead to the occurrence of an epidemic or outbreak, public health authorities need a proper epidemiological investigation, which can guide the further course of action.

Outbreak investigations, an important and challenging component of epidemiology and public health, can help us identify the source of ongoing outbreaks and prevent the occurrence of additional cases. Even when an outbreak is over, findings of epidemiologic and environmental investigations increase our knowledge of a given disease which we can apply for preventing or controlling future outbreaks. Outbreak investigations also provide valuable learning opportunities and foster cooperation between the clinical and public health communities.[106]

Every outbreak needs proper investigations. However, several factors are considered before deciding to investigate or not to investigate an outbreak. These factors could be related to the disease or health condition, the public health system and the community affected.[1] Let's see what all these factors could be;

a) *Disease or health condition related;*
- Severity of the disease
- Rate of its spread to others
- Availability of effective treatment
- Availability of effective prevention and control
- Poor outcome, i.e., disability or death
- New emerging disease (for finding epidemiological details)

b) *Public health system related:*
   - Existence of a trustworthy reporting system
   - Availability of expertise to analyze data from routine reporting or surveillance
   - Availability of financial resources
   - Ability to plan prevention, control and treatment strategies for outbreaks and execute their implementation
   - Synergy with other stakeholders
   - To understand where the existing prevention and control programs failed
   - Administrative and political will

c) *Community or public related;*
   - Large pool of susceptible people
   - Fear related to severe consequences of disease
   - Political considerations
   - Legal reasons
   - Community's apprehension about linkage with poor environmental conditions which may be existing there

Almost every point included in the list above is self-explanatory. However, to understand it further, think and articulate statements on these points giving recommendations to investigate an epidemic as a self-learning exercise. While doing so, imagine you are the local public health authority, and the statement is needed for approval from the director of health services.

Whenever a decision to investigate an outbreak, a cluster or an epidemic, is taken, whatever may be the factors for taking such decision, the investigation should be done following the standard methodological steps. In the ensuing sections, we will see what these steps are.

STEPS INVOLVED IN INVESTIGATING EPIDEMICS

Planning epidemic investigations and executing it methodically ensures that no critical step is missed. You will see that these steps are not isolated ones. Many preparatory steps might be done simultaneously. With the order in which these are mentioned below, it does not mean that they are to be essentially done in the similar sequential manner. Their mention in the list will serve as the necessary checkpoints and at times, may even make us re-think about the strategy, well before the actual investigation is initiated.[106]

1. Prepare for the Field Work

Meticulous preparations for the field work are critical. Those teams which are entirely dedicated to the task of epidemic investigations may find it easy to organize themselves for this task. However, it remains the most important preparatory task for any epidemic investigation team. Preparing in advance will help us get rid of many operational issues that may arise in the field.

Some important elements which should be considered are mentioned below;

Getting information about the cases from local health authorities or through routine reports, or spot maps is critical. Many descriptive details can be worked out from this kind of information.

Gathering information about the geography of the area where field investigation is to be carried out, its access roads, travel time, nearby public health facilities, stay arrangements, etc. are some of the basic details that need to be known in advance. Also, the local environmental and socio-cultural-economic issues are of great significance, and an idea about them in advance would be of help.

Coordination among team members, finalization of investigation structure (through epidemiological investigation forms or software) are also important parts of basic preparatory essentials.

Confirmation of arrangements of vehicles for travel, getting a list of important contact numbers (like local administrators, health authorities, healthcare workers, etc.) help us mitigate lots of operational inconveniences.

In situations where laboratory investigations are required at the field level, all essential preparations should be made. All the laboratories, where investigations are to be carried out, should be identified and their quality standards to be ensured. The investigation team should have good coordination with the laboratory team, and have their advice on sample collection, storage, and its transportation. Proper containers for sample collection should be procured. Timeline from the collection of the samples to their delivery in the laboratory should be discussed with the laboratory staff.

We have recently seen some epidemics of Ebola Virus Disease, which has an average case fatality rate of 50%. The virus is introduced in human population by a certain species of bats. It spreads from one person to another via direct contact with the blood, secretions, organs or other bodily fluids of infected people (through broken skin or mucous membranes), and with surfaces and materials (e.g., bedding, clothing) contaminated with these fluids.

In such situations, healthcare workers or members of an epidemic investigation team should use all essential protective measures for their safety. These measures would depend on the infectivity and routes of transmission of the disease under study. A list in reference to infections like Ebola Virus Disease would include, basic hand hygiene, respiratory hygiene, safe injection practices, use of personal protective equipment (to block splashes or other contact with infected materials) like face protection (a face shield or a medical mask and goggles), a clean, non-sterile long-sleeved gown, and gloves (sterile gloves for some procedures).[107] For many other infectious disease investigations, the team members may need to take specific prophylactic medications or vaccines also.

A well-coordinated team always has a plan of action ready and agreed upon by all members. This helps them avoid field level misunderstandings which may cause unnecessary delays or can even make the investigations less fruitful.[108]

The composition of an epidemic investigation team would depend, to a large extent, on the type of disease being investigated. Looking at some basic composition, as given below, will give us a fair idea about it-

- Epidemiologist
- Public health specialist
- Medical officer
- Concerned specialist (physician, pediatrician, etc.)
- Microbiologist/virologist/pathologist
- Healthcare worker (nursing)
- Laboratory technician (for sample collections, handling, and transport)
- Teams for case finding (local healthcare personnel), information recording
- Other Support staff, like drivers, vehicle mechanics, local guide (if long travel by road in remote interior areas is required).

The list above is just to give an idea, and it will vary from situation to situation.

2. Establish the Existence of An Epidemic

It may sound illogical to say that we must first prepare for the field work and then establish whether an epidemic exists. In actual practice, these steps can go together. When an alert is raised that there is a significant increase in the numbers of cases of a disease in a given area, then epidemiological investigations should be conducted. By *'establishing the existence of an epidemic'* it implies that the data on the basis of which the alert is raised should be carefully examined and analyzed. Many times, observed numbers of the disease appear to have increased over the routinely expected numbers because the reporting system is strengthened or surveillance has improved, or the denominator has undergone a reduction in size recently (e.g., mass migration of people, out of the area, for earning livelihoods) or diagnosis made was wrong. The epidemiologists need to figure it out and come to the conclusion that the observed cases are genuinely more than the expected numbers.

Whether it is an unexpected clustering of cases in a small localized area, an outbreak in small geography or an epidemic in a comparatively wider geography, a thorough and careful investigation is warranted. When in the initial stages, if any particular incident does not fit into standard definitions of a cluster, an outbreak or an epidemic, but it still suspected to pose a serious public health risk, then proper epidemiological investigations are paramount.[106, 108]

3. Verifying the Diagnosis

Here also, we need to note that establishing the existence of an epidemic and verifying the diagnosis may go on parallelly. Verification of diagnosis is a critical step as the entire set of actions to find out epidemiological details, giving correct treatment, implementing appropriate prevention and control strategies, are linked to establishing the correct diagnosis.[1, 109]

For establishing a correct clinical diagnosis, the team of epidemiologists relies on clinical and laboratory investigations. Epidemiologists, public health experts, and clinicians would need to personally see and examine some cases, and take a detailed history. Also, in this exercise appropriate laboratory investigations will be required. Depending on the diagnosis which is likely, these investigations can be biochemical, immunological, bacteriological, virologic, or any other as relevant.

For checking consistency with diagnosis and for developing a case definition, many times epidemiologists use clinical features frequency distribution. If, say, twenty cases are examined initially, and their clinical features are put in a frequency distribution. The resultant distribution trend will help epidemiologists in checking the consistency of clinical features with the diagnosis that is being considered. Let's assume; in the initial examination of twenty cases in an outbreak, we find that 90% of cases have fever 101 deg. F or more, developed a maculopapular rash on 3rd or 4th day of illness which fades away after 4-5 days of appearance, and there is accompanying cough and cold in 80% cases. Then, these points are worth considering for developing a working case definition for the epidemiological investigations.[106, 108]

4. Develop a Working Case Definition

A working case definition is a standard set of criteria, used for deciding whether an individual should be classified as having the disease or health condition in reference. We need a working case definition to ensure that uniform criteria are applied in identifying the cases. When cases are searched actively over a wider geographical area, this would require the deployment of many healthcare workers or volunteers. Not having common criteria, would result in confusion among them about the cases to be selected or excluded. Secondly, in a working case definition, we use a set of simple and obviously understandable criteria that would not require an expert clinical examination by clinicians for confirming every case. A working case definition for epidemic investigation purpose differs from a clinical definition. The former uses simple criteria that are stated clearly, leaves no ambiguity and is easy to use. It should also be applicable in a standard manner by different people under different circumstances.[1, 106]

Definitions used in clinical settings are backed by clinical judgment made thorough clinical examinations, and laboratory investigations. The standard case definitions used for surveillance are a set of standard criteria for classifying whether a person has a particular disease, syndrome, or other health condition. Many of the case definitions, specifically those which are used for national or worldwide surveillance, are adopted as standard ones to ensure national and international comparability. Use of such standardized definitions ensures that cases are identified applying uniform standards, irrespective of who identifies them or in which place these are identified.[1]

The case definitions developed for outbreak investigations are contextualized to the local situation. These definitions always have clearly spelled out clinical criteria, and also some laboratory criteria at times. Outbreak case definitions may also have some restrictions regarding time place and person. For example, if we say that *'child under 15 years of age with clinical criteria'*, then it becomes an age restriction. Similarly, we can put time restriction such as *'onset within last 06 months'* and place restrictions by saying *'residing within the district for last 06 months'*.

Most of the times, in outbreak investigations, we need some degree of flexibility to pick up a case on even slightest of suspicion. This is required and is beneficial to leave no chance. So, we use appropriate criteria in the definitions that help us categorize cases as *suspected*, *probable* or *confirmed*. We will consider an example of malaria here to understand this clearly;

Clinical Description of Malaria:

Malaria should be considered in any patient who presents with Fever and any 2 of the following.

- Chills, Sweating, Jaundice, Spleen enlargement (splenomegaly)
- Convulsions, Coma, shock, pulmonary edema and death may be associated with severe cases

Laboratory Criteria for Diagnosis

- Demonstration of Malaria Parasite in blood film

OR

- Positive Rapid Diagnostic Test for Malaria

Case Classification

- *Suspected*: Any Case of Fever (in an area where malaria exists)
- *Probable:* A case that meets the clinical case definition
- *Confirmed:* A suspected/probable case that is laboratory- confirmed (A laboratory-confirmed case does not need to meet the clinical case definition.) [110, 111]

Public health authorities, in order to identify every possible case, use a sensitive case definition. Such definitions include almost all cases which truly have the given disease. However, by using such definitions, many other cases of illnesses that are somewhat similar to the illness being investigated, are also picked up.

When it comes to studying causation of an outbreak of a disease, investigators use a strict or specific definition. They would want that any individual included in the study truly has the disease under study (no false case is picked up) and any person not having the disease is not included as a case.[106]

Hopefully, now the importance of working case definition is clear.

5. Systematic Case Finding and Information Recording

In an outbreak, the cases coming to the notice of health authorities may be those who have either self-reported or were found by neighbors or other community members. The cases noticed above are not the entire picture of the situation. The entire picture would include other cases also who could not either self-report or come to anyone's notice. For finding such cases, an active effort by local healthcare personnel is needed. Every healthcare person, deployed for the task of case finding will have to use the case definitions, developed for that outbreak, as the uniform yardstick to identify the cases. The cases would be found either in the community, or they would report to nearby healthcare facilities. Therefore, measures of case finding should be directed towards both, the community as well as healthcare facilities (and practitioners).

Public health authorities should send detailed information about the outbreak to all healthcare facilities, both public and private. All practitioners and health facilities should promptly intimate about any case that visits them. This is passive surveillance for the cases.

Local healthcare authorities should launch an intensive search for cases in the community. This may involve house to house search in the area affected by the outbreak. This is active surveillance. Each of the cases detected should be subjected to the basic investigations first. Details like personal habits, specific exposures, contact with people, the progression of illness and similarly other relevant information can be found out from a detailed history obtained from them. From clinical examinations, we can find out about specific clinical features, their order of onset, and other clinical signs.

Another important source of case reporting is a well-informed community. Therefore, it is important to communicate widely about the outbreak in an appropriate manner, without creating any panic.

For every case detected, following set of information should be recorded;

Identification Details: Such as name, address with landmarks, contact information

Demographic and Risk Factor Details: Like age, sex, occupation, information about race, family details, specific risk factor details, exposure to possible risk factors, etc

Clinical Information: Signs, symptoms, onset of illness, its progression, history of any treatment received, history of contact, investigation details, etc.[108]

Once we get a complete picture, we should start plotting cases against the time of occurrence to get what is known as an **epidemic curve**. This process of plotting cases on the epidemic curve should be continued as the situation keeps evolving even when the investigations are going on.

Epidemic curve helps epidemiologists to get some idea about the type of epidemic, whether it is a point source, propagated or intermittent source. It also helps them understand the magnitude of the outbreak and about its phase, i.e., rising, stationary or declining.[1]

In the sample curve below in figure 36, cases occurring day wise are plotted. For diseases that have a very short incubation period and where it is important to subdivide a day into two halves or four quarters further, we may accordingly prepare the epidemic curve.

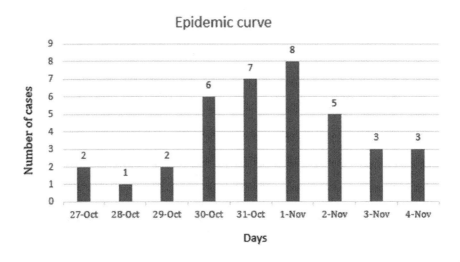

Figure 36: Example of an epidemic curve

6. Working Out Descriptive Epidemiologic Details

Once the relevant information as stated above is collected, the next step is to systematically organize this information and describe key findings. This includes distribution of the disease under study, in terms of time, place and persons. In other words, we work out descriptive epidemiologic details.[106] Performing descriptive epidemiologic exercise at this stage has manifold advantages;

- We can understand the basic characterization of an outbreak through time, person and place distribution.

- These descriptive details help us understand which are the worst affected locations, population groups, and also the timings of occurrence. This information is useful for health authorities to intensify prevention and control efforts, through appropriate channelization of resources.

- Descriptive details provide important leads to the etiology of the disease, also towards risk factors, source, mode of transmission, which are useful for formulating the hypothesis of causation.

We know, from our descriptive epidemiology chapter, about organizing information to understand time, place and person distribution, and benefits of doing so. The updated epidemic curve should also be referred to at every stage of the epidemic investigation. This exercise, of updating the epidemic curve and referring to it, should go on even after completion of the outbreak investigations.

Place and person distribution details provide valuable clues to the epidemiologists, which are very useful in formulating a hypothesis. For example, if the affected people are those who ate something from a common eatery then it points towards some food born etiology. If the sufferers are those who had unsafe sex with a common commercial sex worker, then the disease could be a sexually transmitted one. Likewise, if we notice cases of a disease with respiratory symptoms, in an area which is close to an industry emitting heavy air pollutants, then we get a clue pointing towards the probable cause.[108]

7. Formulating Hypothesis

Information analyzed from preceding steps helps us in formulating a hypothesis. Also, epidemiologists hold an in-person discussion with affected individuals, to gather information regarding behaviors, exposures, food habits, travel in and out from the affected area, associated illness (if any), occupation factors- if relevant, family level determinants, etc. Many times, personal discussions can be very helpful and provide valuable clues for hypothesis formulation.[106] Detailed history and clinical examination also provide important inputs that help in formulating the hypothesis.

As discussed in the point about descriptive epidemiology above, descriptive details are critically important. We get highly valuable indications from the pattern of persons getting affected or special characteristics associated with the places that show a high number of cases, or the time distribution patterns. For example, if the time distribution or epidemic curve shows a single peak that lasted for a short duration, showing the rapid rise and gradual decline, in all probabilities, it is indicating towards a disease of short incubation period that has originated from a point source. In a point-source epidemic, all the cases occur within one incubation period. If the duration of exposure is prolonged, the epidemic is called a **continuous common-source epidemic**, and the epidemic curve has a plateau instead of a peak. An intermittent common-source epidemic (in which exposure to the causative agent is sporadic over time) usually produces an irregularly jagged epidemic curve reflecting the intermittence and duration of exposure and the number of persons exposed. A **propagated epidemic** — that spreads from person-to-person with increasing numbers of cases in each generation of contacts— should have a series of progressively taller peaks one incubation period apart. However, if we do not have idea about the complete situation, in its early stages, we may not find these classic patterns. A solid hypothesis requires all these points to be considered along with clinical details or any investigation results that are available. It is always necessary to evaluate the hypothesis after it is proposed.[108]

8. Evaluating the Hypothesis

Once, a hypothesis is formulated, it is checked for its reasonability and probability. This evaluation is done with the help of clinical investigations, laboratory investigations, the study of local environmental factors, and epidemiological methods.

There are situations when clinical, laboratory or environmental findings are sufficient to support the hypothesis. In such situations, where a clear-cut evidence is not established, analytical epidemiological methods are applied to evaluate the hypothesis. Figure 37 shows a decision making tree to help us remember the course of action in different situations in this regard.

Investigating an Epidemic

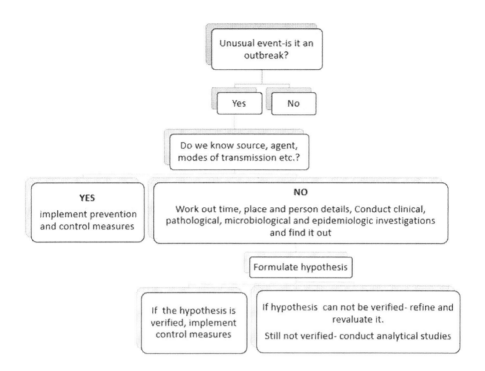

Figure 37: Decision-making tree for epidemic investigations

Under situations when the hypothesis could not be verified, the basic question that needs to be answered through this approach of applying analytical methods is, whether the observed occurrence is more in the exposed individuals as compared to that which is routinely expected in non-exposed. If it is more in the exposed group, then the next checkpoint is to ascertain the fact that this difference is not merely by chance. This is done by using statistical methods like tests of significance. The epidemiological methods that are applied are either retrospective cohort or case-control studies. Epidemiologists analyze relative and attributable risks to understand the role of the key suspected factor in disease causation and degree of its association with the outcome.[106, 108] For detailed steps in these analytical methods, please refer back to the chapter on analytical epidemiology.

9. Reconsideration, Refinement or Re-Evaluation of Hypothesis

Many times, the epidemiologists, when not finding any substantial supportive evidence, relook at the proposed hypothesis, carry out need-based refinements as per evidence from the field findings. In some circumstances, even this fails to generate concrete supportive evidence for the proposed hypothesis. Often, under this scenario, multiple analytical epidemiologic studies are required to ascertain the cause-effect association.

There are also incidents where detailed re-discussion with affected individuals, their family members, and friends provided important clues which investigators could not discover at first instance. Also, discussions with the local healthcare workers can give us some valuable information to reinforce the hypothesis proposed initially. Accordingly, the epidemiologists refine hypothesis and then re-evaluate it to check its reasonability and probability.[108]

10. Compare and Verify with Laboratory Findings

This is the final checkpoint before epidemiologists recommend actions. The final hypothesis should be verified with the evidence generated by the laboratory studies. If there is a mismatch, then they will have to revisit the hypothesis. Laboratory findings can be of specific biomarkers, any pathological test such as the culture of samples from cases, or testing of vehicles like food, water, milk or any environmental condition assessment like contamination of drinking water source, air quality standards, etc.

Once, the proposed hypothesis corroborates with the laboratory or environmental investigations' results; we treat the hypothesis as verified and confirmed.[108]

11. Implementing Prevention and Control Measures

It is important to understand that the general prevention and control measures are instituted on getting the first evidence of the existence of an outbreak. Though, disease-specific prevention and control measures are implemented once its diagnosis is confirmed. As we know, one of the core strategies in prevention and control measures' implementation and their acceptance by the community, is proper communication. Clear communication about the disease is critical. It should be done in a way that does not cause panic among people or stigmatize those who are affected.

Specific prevention and control strategies would have different components for different diseases. It would include elements like vaccinating susceptible people, giving chemoprophylaxis to susceptible persons where relevant, isolating affected individuals, controlling environmental factors where relevant, cutting or reducing transmission through vectors or vehicles, eliminating or controlling risk factors, ensuring proper treatment to those affected, etc.

The public health authorities implement prevention and control activities. Therefore, it is a recommended practice for the outbreak investigation team to work in full coordination with the local health authorities and health workers too. Slightest miscommunication and resulting misunderstanding can create mistrust within the affected community, and it will adversely impact the cooperation that community members offer in the entire process.[106]

12. Start or Maintain Surveillance

In an outbreak, cluster or epidemic, assuming that the number of cases would no longer rise again, will be a huge mistake. Therefore, it is essential to ensure that there is a system of surveillance, both active and passive, that is in place. On the basis of findings from epidemiological investigations, a standard surveillance definition should be adopted. All healthcare workers, in the affected and adjoining areas, should be oriented, so that surveillance for the cases goes on uniformly, using the same definition. Also, a prompt case reporting system should be activated so that there is no delay in case reporting. Keeping the affected communities well informed about case reporting is very useful. Alert community members report many cases in the situations of epidemics.

For ensuring that passive surveillance at the health facilities, both public and private, remains effective, a proper briefing of all healthcare personnel should be conducted by respective facility in-charges. Here again, uniformity in the information disseminated needs to be ensured. Hence, the use of standard information, education, communication (IEC) material is recommended to all facilities.

13. Report Findings and Share Recommendations

Clear communication about the final findings and recommendations guides the future steps meant for effective prevention and control. It is critical to mention all key factors that played a part in the occurrence of the outbreak. This helps health authorities and other stakeholders to develop and implement an effective, well-coordinated, multipronged approach to contain the disease.

For better understanding, avoiding any possibility of confusion, the ideal approach is to hold detailed discussions with public health and administrative authorities, also involving key stakeholders having a role to play in prevention and control work.

An exhaustive written report is essential for records and reference and should always be shared with all concerned authorities.

 Points to Remember

- Different factors that help us decide about investigating an epidemic.
- What all things we should keep in mind while preparing to investigate an epidemic.
- How is existence of an epidemic confirmed.
- Importance of verifying the diagnosis.
- Importance of developing a working case definition.
- Systematic case findings.
- Benefits that 'working out descriptive details' provide to us.
- What do we mean by an etiological hypothesis.
- Why evaluating the hypothesis is important.
- Role descriptive epidemiologic details play in helping public health system to plan and prioritize prevention and control measures in an epidemic scenario.
- Importance of proper reporting of investigation findings.

CHAPTER
12

PUBLIC HEALTH SURVEILLANCE

Learning Objectives

- ❖ Understand the concept of surveillance.
- ❖ Know what are the key characteristics of surveillance.
- ❖ How does a surveillance system work (its core functions).
- ❖ Know about basic types of surveillance.
- ❖ Learn about some objective based categories of surveillance.

The word surveillance is derived from two French words, *sur*-meaning 'over' and *veiller*-meaning 'to watch'. From the word itself we can guess it has something to do with being watchful for something. We have often come across statements like *'police have installed surveillance cameras'* or *'the army is conducting surveillance in the area to detect suspicious antinational elements.'* As per Merriam-Webster's dictionary, surveillance means 'to closely and continuously watch one or more persons for the purpose of direction, supervision or control'.[112] According to the Cambridge dictionary of English (online), the word means 'careful watching of a person or place, especially by the police or army, because of a crime that has happened or is expected'.[113]

The concept of surveillance, when applied to public health, means keeping a watch over the frequency of disease occurrence or its pattern in an ongoing manner.

WHO defines Public health surveillance as the continuous, systematic collection, analysis and interpretation of health-related data needed for the planning, implementation, and evaluation of public health practice. Such surveillance can:

> Serve as an early warning system for impending public health emergencies;

> Document the impact of an intervention, or track progress towards specified goals; and

> Monitor and clarify the epidemiology of health problems, to allow priorities to be set and to inform public health policy and strategies.[114]

When we talk about health-related data in the context of surveillance, we mean disease, health status or risk factors related data in any given population. Data gathered through surveillance is always used for facilitating prevention and control of given disease or health outcome or behavior.

Larger objectives of the information generated from disease surveillance, also linked to prevention, control, and treatment, are

- To identify the persons affected by the disease so that they can be treated adequately and promptly.
- To guide prevention and control strategies to protect other susceptible persons.
- To understand what impact existing prevention and control program is having on the disease occurrence.[115]

Since surveillance is not a standalone activity and is always linked to prevention and control, we need to have clearly spelled out process details like case definition, mode and frequency of data collection, how will it be compiled and analyzed, and in what way it would be used for reinforcing prevention and control.

Effective communicable disease control relies on effective response systems, and effective response systems rely on effective disease surveillance. A functional surveillance system is essential in providing information for action on priority communicable diseases; it is a crucial instrument for public health decision-making in all countries.[116]

KEY CHARACTERISTICS OF SURVEILLANCE

Some of the important characteristics of surveillance that are critical and are always kept at the forefront are:

Timeliness: As we have discussed that any surveillance activity in public health, always has linkages with prevention and control activities for the disease concerned. Therefore, it is essential that it is conducted in a timely manner.[115, 117, 118]

Representativeness: coverage of the surveillance activity should be such that it gives us a comprehensive picture of the evolving temporal trend (time-related) of the disease. For example, surveillance for poliomyelitis conducted across nations gave us the trend over time and this became the basis of certifying individual countries if they achieved polio-free status.[115, 117, 118]

Sensitivity: Sensitivity in surveillance refers to the proportion of actual cases in a population that are detected and notified through the system. Sensitivity is particularly important in an early warning system designed to detect outbreaks. Surveillance methods adopted should be sensitive so that it identifies affected individuals and thus can facilitate their treatment. This way, relevant prevention and control measures are implemented in response to detection of cases. For example, detection of cases of poliomyelitis, under ongoing polio eradication initiative, is based on finding cases with acute flaccid paralysis, which invariably captures all paralytic poliomyelitis cases. Undoubtedly, the surveillance criteria used (acute flaccid paralysis) is a proxy-criteria for poliomyelitis (syndromic surveillance approach) and it captures some non-poliomyelitis cases, but these are excluded through laboratory confirmation tests.[115, 118]

Specificity: The surveillance method used should be such that the persons without the disease are excluded. In other words, specificity refers to the proportion of persons without the disease, who are considered by the surveillance system as not having the disease. As we know, from the public health angle, in case of surveillance for infectious diseases, it is acceptable to have few false positive cases rather than to miss even a small number of cases. But, very low specificity would result in the surveillance system indicating many "false" outbreaks, and the staff would be spending a lot of resources to verify and investigate.[115] To take care of such an eventuality, some mechanism for confirming the cases that are picked up using standard definition, through means of appropriate laboratory investigations, is integrated in a surveillance system, wherever needed.

For example, in acute flaccid paralysis surveillance for poliomyelitis, sometimes, cases of diseases other than poliomyelitis, that may also cause acute flaccid paralysis, like Guillain Barré Syndrome, traumatic neuritis, transverse myelitis, etc. were also picked up. However, with laboratory investigation (isolation of poliovirus from stool samples), it is easy to exclude them.

Besides these critical characteristics as mentioned above, there are some other characteristics also that are important and should be factored into the surveillance strategy. These are;

Acceptability: Acceptability of a system is a reflection of the willingness of the surveillance staff to implement the system, and of the end users to accept and use the data generated by the system. In simplest words, this means how easy is the surveillance system's operation.[118] By evaluation of the acceptability of a surveillance system, we come to know whether the team members implementing it or those supporting the system, view it as appropriate to the requirements. In cases where the system is found to be inappropriate, suggestions should be made for improving it to make it more acceptable to the implementers and end users of the data.[115]

Flexibility: Flexibility refers to the ability of the system to adapt to changing needs such as the removal or inclusion of additional diseases, modification of the reporting frequency, data requirement needs, etc. In other words, this would mean how quickly the system can adapt to changes.[118] The system should also be flexible enough to shift from serving the needs for outbreak detection to providing for outbreak response and control.[115]

Positive predictive value: It means that the method used should be able to clearly identify a high percentage of those individuals who have the disease, as true positive cases. The number of those without disease reported as positives (false positives) should be the minimum possible. In reference to epidemics, this also means that the surveillance system should correctly identify actual epidemics. A method or system not able to do so will result in unnecessary wastage of time, money and other resources.

Quality: The quality of the surveillance system is defined by attributes such as completeness, timeliness, usefulness, sensitivity, positive predictive value (PPV), specificity, representativeness, simplicity, flexibility, acceptability, and reliability. These individual attributes have been discussed in preceding paragraphs.

Validity: This refers to ability of the method or system to generate information or data that it is supposed to generate.[115]

Stability: This indicates that the personnel, equipment, other resources and the entire system of surveillance is well positioned and it operates as per laid down standards. Also, the data generated is readily available for the public health system to guide its response.

Simplicity: Simplicity refers to the structure of the system and the ease of implementation. In other words, it indicates how easy is the system's operation. Any surveillance strategy which is in use, not only should fulfill important criteria as mentioned above in preceding paragraphs but should also retain its simplicity. Regarding implementation, the amount and type of information collected, ease of collection, compilation, analysis, reporting, and ease of using the reporting system are the key factors that should be considered. In relation to the structure of the system, the simplicity of information flow from its point of generation to the end users, and complementarity of different components to one another are important criteria for consideration.[115, 118]

CORE FUNCTIONS OF A SURVEILLANCE SYSTEM[115, 118]

Any surveillance is a part of a larger network of activities and responses. This entire framework constitutes the surveillance system. In the following points, we will see what the core functions are which a larger surveillance system performs;

Case detection: Identifying cases of a disease or its outbreak is the pivotal function. Case detection can be done through the formal healthcare system, private healthcare institutions or practitioners (also includes the alternative system of indigenous medicine practitioners) or from community networks through volunteers, grassroots level health workers or community members.

Case registration: As we know completeness of information for each case detected is crucial. Therefore, detected cases are registered using a standard register or a case details form. Each case is assigned a unique identification number for further reference and tracking.

Case confirmation: Ground level surveillance personnel identify cases using the standard case definition. However, a confirmatory clinical assessment is required in cases which have a confusing presentation. To cater to this need, surveillance systems usually engage concerned super-specialists for their expert opinion on such cases. For the final confirmation, the system relies on the laboratory facilities in its network. Whether it's single or multiple, laboratories should operate using the standard guidelines as required by the surveillance system. Also, there should be a system of quality assurance and control, through internal and external quality control approaches, which ensures high reliability of the results from the participating laboratories.

Reporting: Surveillance systems have clearly defined reporting guidelines. Prompt reporting of cases, reporting of the occurrence of an epidemic, besides routine periodic reporting, are vitally important reporting activities. Different national projects have different reporting guidelines as per their requirements.

Data analysis and interpretation: In order to facilitate continuous vigil over the disease in reference, the surveillance systems need resources and expertise to carry out data analysis and interpretation at the required frequency. Some disease may require a day to day interpretation whereas there are others which may need a weekly or monthly analysis and interpretation of the data generated. This helps public health system to get timely epidemic alerts or reinforce existing surveillance strategy, wherever required.

Preparedness for epidemic response and other public health actions: Surveillance systems generate data that constantly indicate towards changes in disease situation. Rising numbers of cases require public health preparedness for epidemic response. To address such an eventuality, the system needs to have an appropriate operational plan ready and also, a reserve pool of skilled personnel and required supplies such as vaccines or medications. Availability of adequate hospitalization and isolation (infectious diseases) capacity is also an area that should be factored into the preparedness plans.

Epidemic response evaluation and control: Generally, elements to evaluate the quality and completeness of an epidemic response are integrated into surveillance systems. This helps improve subsequent responses.

Feedback: It is mentioned at the end of the list but is critical for timeliness and completeness of public health response. All those who have direct control over the public health operation and also those directing surveillance operations need reliable feedback. Regular, clear and complete feedback based on the data generated through surveillance activities, and also on the basis of supervisory or monitoring visits is an essential function of surveillance systems.

BASIC TYPES OF SURVEILLANCE

We can classify public health surveillance into three key types. These are;

1. Passive Surveillance
2. Active Surveillance
3. Sentinel Surveillance

Passive Surveillance[118]

Under this type of surveillance, health practitioners, healthcare workers, investigating laboratories or hospitals and other healthcare institutions voluntarily report cases of the disease under surveillance to the designated health authorities or the surveillance project authorities. It is important to ensure a uniform understanding of what to report across people and institutions participating in passive surveillance, through written guidelines or discussions. The information-set which participating personnel or institutions are required to provide is simple and direct. There is no active search for cases carried out by the surveillance personnel, either in the communities or institutions.[119]

The passive surveillance system is the least expensive of all surveillance methods and most commonly used for vaccine-preventable diseases in many countries. Also, through this approach, it is possible to cover very wide geography, utilizing the existing network of healthcare providers and institutions. Since a large number of personnel and institutions participate, sometimes it becomes difficult to ensure completeness and timeliness of reporting. However, through effective feedback on these issues, participating personnel and institutions can be made to improve upon these aspects of reporting.

Active Surveillance[118]

This type of surveillance provides most accurate information, but it requires more resources. The surveillance project engages trained personnel who actively visit health facilities or populations and gather information about the disease or health events. This provides most accurate information promptly but is an expensive approach.[119]

When the health systems effectively work towards elimination or eradication of a particular infectious disease, its cases may show a gradually declining trend in numbers. Even in such situations, when the numbers of cases are declining, ensuring completeness of reporting is important. Also, delay in case detection has to be avoided, as prompt control measures may be required in response to the cases detected. Such situations require active surveillance to be in place. For example, under polio eradication initiative, robust active surveillance was put in place to help move countries and regions towards polio elimination and then to polio eradication phase.

Active surveillance approach also recommends that surveillance field personnel follow a system of 'nil reporting' in a situation when no new case is detected in an area under surveillance. This helps in avoiding the situation of missing out a case.

Sentinel Surveillance[118]

Public health system requires a detailed, high-quality data on diseases. Such details cannot be obtained through passive surveillance and even through active surveillance by healthcare field personnel unless specialist personnel are engaged. In geographical areas that have a higher occurrence of a given disease, those institutions which are likely to see many cases of the disease in reference, are selected as sentinel sites. As these sites, which are generally some high-volume hospitals or other healthcare institutions, have healthcare specialists, obtaining detailed information about individual cases from them does not pose any difficulty. As the diagnostic facilities and expertise are also available in these centers, the case reporting is more accurate. However, it should be noted that these sentinel sites represent a sample based surveillance, covering the population sample reporting to that sentinel site for their healthcare needs. Therefore, due care should be taken to extrapolate estimates derived from sentinel surveillance to the general population.

Sentinel surveillance is excellent for detection of public health problems that are commonly found. This approach is not suitable for the disease of rare occurrence, new emerging diseases, as these conditions require a timely and active search in the susceptible population.[119]

CATEGORIZATION OF SURVEILLANCE STRATEGIES BASED ON SPECIFIC SITUATIONS

Some of the surveillance strategies have been devised to meet specific public health objectives of disease detection and control. Key categories are as below;

Laboratory-based surveillance: In case of infectious diseases, this approach is highly valuable. If any laboratory under a surveillance network, detects a pathogenic organism which has potential to cause an epidemic, it is required to be reported to a notified surveillance or public health authority. The sentinel site, from which such a sample is received, can provide necessary case details that are useful for reinforcing control measures.

Laboratory-based surveillance can provide early warning signals that help detect an outbreak. It can be helpful in outbreak response evaluation during the outbreak. This approach is of value for disease trend monitoring, intervention evaluation and also for monitoring progress towards control objective once the outbreak subsides. Quality control standards are an essential part to ensure uniformity of performance standards for participating laboratories.[120] Establishing a laboratory-based surveillance system will need expertise, resources, facilities, and training. A central public health reference laboratory is essential for oversight at the participating laboratories for quality assurance, quality control and other technical support.[119]

Syndromic surveillance: This strategy focusses on syndromes rather than specific diseases.[118] The syndromic surveillance system is an active or passive system that uses case definitions based entirely on clinical features without any clinical or laboratory diagnosis. A simple example would be, collecting the number of cases of diarrhoea rather than cases of cholera, or "rash illness" rather than measles.[119] In this reference, with the term syndrome, we mean a group of signs and symptoms utilized for identifying the cases. For example, fever with chills, fever with rashes, cough with shortness of breath, fever with burning micturition, etc. are some most commonly used syndromic groups. There can be a variety of such combinations depending on the disease conditions to be watched.

Based on syndromic surveillance, we can identify potential cases when they report to a health facility for seeking medical care, which can be a few days before the actual diagnosis is made. Under this strategy, some syndrome is monitored as a proxy for the given disease-like looking for acute flaccid paralysis to detect cases of poliomyelitis.

The primary goal of syndromic surveillance is to give indications of an unusual increase in illnesses, much earlier than traditional surveillance would give. However, being based on suspected syndromic combinations, the strategy is less specific and would include many individuals who do not actually have the disease.[1]

Integrated surveillance: A combination of active and passive systems using a single infrastructure that gathers information about multiple diseases or behaviors which are of interest to several intervention programs. Such systems, if they are health facility-based, may gather information on multiple infectious diseases and injuries.[119]

Integrated surveillance strategy is more cost-effective than having isolated disease-specific surveillance programs. Even in a situation where there are multiple vertical disease-specific surveillance programs in existence, control response is mediated through a common public health department. Sometimes, few specific diseases are accorded higher priority either because of international requirements or due to local reasons. Resultingly, the respective surveillance programs get more attention (funds, personnel, supplies) and start performing in a better way. In contrast to this, there are some disease surveillance programs which underperform because of lesser attention they get.

Integration is a solution for such discrimination. An integrated approach to communicable disease surveillance encompasses all surveillance activities in a country. It works as a common public service which carries out many functions while it uses similar structures, processes, and personnel. The benefit of integrating also goes to the surveillance activities that are not so well developed in any given aspect. Here, the surveillance programs that are well developed may act as driving forces for strengthening other surveillance activities, offering possible synergies and common resources.[116]

Integrated disease surveillance program in India (IDSP) is an example which is worth referring to, for further understanding of integrated approach.[121]

 Points to Remember

- Concept of surveillance.
- Key characteristics of surveillance.
- Core functions a surveillance system performs.
- Basic types of surveillance (active, passive and sentinel surveillance).
- Objective based categories of surveillance like laboratory, syndromic and integrated surveillance.

References

1. **CDC.** *Introduction to epidemiology, 3rd edition-Department of Health and Human Services, Centre for Disease Control and Prevention (CDC).* Atlanta: CDC, 2006. pp. 6.25-6.28.
2. **Last, JM.** *A dictionary of epidemiology.* [ed.] Last JM. s.l.: Oxford University Press, 2001.
3. **JM, Last.** *A dictionary of epidemiology.* s.l.: Oxford university press, 2001. pp. 53, 78, 80.
4. **CDC.** Centre for Disease Control and Prevention, Yellow Book. s.l.: Department of Health and Human Services, Centre for Disease Control and Prevention (CDC), 2018.
5. **Bonita R, Beaglehole R., Kjellstrom T.** *Basic Epidemiology.* s.l.: WHO, 2006. p. 19.
6. **CSDH.** Closing the gap in a generation: health equity through action on the social determinants of health. Final Report of the Commission on Social Determinants of Health. *www.who.int.* [Online] 2008. http://apps.who.int/iris/bitstream/10665/43943/1/9789241563703_eng.pdf.
7. *The uses of 'uses of epidemiology'.* **Smith, George Davey.** 2001, International Journal of Epidemiology, Vol. 30, pp. 1146-1155.
8. **Beaglehole R, Bonita R,.** Public health at crossroads: achievements and prospects. s.l.: Cambridge University Press, 2004.
9. **NCI.** www.cancer.gov (National Cancer Institute at National Institute of Health). *www.cancer.gov.* [Online] 2017. https://www.cancer.gov/about-cancer/causes-prevention/risk/tobacco/cessation-fact-sheet#q2.
10. **Sackett, D.L., Haynes, R.B., Buyatt, G.H., and Tugwell, P. (cited by Roger Detels, M.D., Epidemiology: the foundation of public health M.S.).** Epidemiology: the foundation of public health. *UCLA Fielding School of Public Health.* [Online] 1991. http://www.ph.ucla.edu/epi/faculty/detels/PH150/Detels_Epidemiology.pdf.
11. **WHO.** World Health Organization. [Online] 2010. http://www.who.int/immunization/sage/Polio_GRADing_tables.pdf.

12. *Accelerated progress to reduce under-5 mortality in India.* **Bhan, M.K.** 4, October 2013, The Lancet. Global Health, Vol. 1, pp. 172-3.

13. *Causes of neonatal and child mortality in India: a nationally representative mortality survey.* **MIllion Death Study Collaborators, Bassani DG, Kumar R, Awasthi S, Morris SK, Paul VK, Shet A, Ram U, Gaffey MF, Black RE, Jha P.** 9755, 2010, The Lancet, Vol. 376, pp. 1853-60.

14. *Diarrheal diseases among children in India: Current scenario and future perspectives.* **Lakshminarayanan S, Jayalakshmy R.** 1, 2015, Journal of natural science, biology and medicine, Vol. 6, pp. 24-28.

15. **Cochrane, AL.** Effectiveness and Efficacy, Random Reflections on Health Services. [book auth.] Nuffield Trust. London: Royal Society of Medicine Press, 1999.

16. *Genetic epidemiology.* **Kaprio, Jaakko.** 1257, 2000, The BMJ, Vol. 320.

17. *The science and art of molecular epidemiology.* **Slattery, M L.** 10, s.l.: group.bmj.com, 2002, Journal of Epidemiology & Community Health, Vol. 56.

18. **Johns Hopkins Medicine.** Johns Hopkins Medicine-General Internal Medicine-Pharmacoepidemiology Research. *Johns Hopkins Medicine.* [Online] 2017. https://www.hopkinsmedicine.org/gim/research/content/pharmacoepi.html.

19. **NLM.** MeSH (Medical Subject Headings)-NLM controlled vocabulary thesaurus. *National Institute of Health.* [Online] 2008. https://meshb.nlm.nih.gov/record/ui?name=Endemic%20Diseases.

20. MeSH (Medical Subject Headings)- NLM controlled vocabulary thesaurus used for indexing articles for PubMed. *The National Center for Biotechnology Information -National Institute of Health/National Library of Medicine.* [Online] 2011. https://www.ncbi.nlm.nih.gov/mesh/?term=pandemic.

21. **WHO.** World Health Organization. *World Health Organization-frequently asked questions-What is the WHO definition of health?* [Online] 1948. http://www.who.int/suggestions/faq/en/.

22. **CDC.** Principles of Epidemiology in Public Health Practice, Third Edition, An Introduction to Applied Epidemiology and Biostatistics. *Centre for Disease Prevention and Control.* [Online] 2012. https://www.cdc.gov/ophss/csels/dsepd/ss1978/lesson3/section2.html.

23. **OECD.** GLOSSARY OF STATISTICAL TERMS. *ORGANIZATION FOR ECONOMIC COOPERATION AND DEVELOPMENT.* [Online] 2006. https://stats.oecd.org/glossary/detail.asp?ID=2081.

24. **WHO.** THE GLOBAL BURDEN OF DISEASE-2004 UPDATE. World Health Organization. Geneva: s.n., 2008. p. 28.

25. **NIH.** PubMed Health-National Center for Biotechnology Information (NCBI) at the U.S. National Library of Medicine (NLM). *U.S. National Library of Medicine.* [Online] 2017. https://www.ncbi.nlm.nih.gov/pubmedhealth/PMHT0029373/.

26. **OECD.** GLOSSARY OF STATISTICAL TERMS. *ORGANIZATION FOR ECONOMIC COOPERATION AND DEVELOPMENT.* [Online] 2013. https://stats.oecd.org/glossary/detail.asp?ID=491.

27. **WHO.** Global Health Observatory (GHO). *World Health Organization.* [Online] 2017. http://www.who.int/gho/epidemic_diseases/cholera/situation_trends_case_fatality_ratio/en/.

28. World Health Organization-WHO Statistical Information System (WHOSIS). *WHO Statistical Information System (WHOSIS).* [Online] 2006. http://www.who.int/whosis/whostat2006DefinitionsAndMetadata.pdf?ua=1.

29. **DHS.** The DHS Program- Demographic and Health Surveys- United States Agency for International Development (USAID). [Online] 2017. https://dhsprogram.com/topics/Infant-and-Child-Mortality.cfm.

30. **WHO.** Health statistics and information systems-Global Reference List of 100 Core Health Indicators, 2015. *World Health Organization.* [Online] 2015. http://www.who.int/healthinfo/indicators/2015/chi_2015_26_mortality_under5.pdf.

31. **DHS.** The DHS Program- Demographic and Health Surveys- United States Agency for International Development (USAID). [Online] 2017. https://dhsprogram.com/Topics/Infant-and-Child-Mortality.cfm.

32. **Mwale, Macleod W.** *Malawi Demographic and Health Survey 2004 (Chapter 8-Infant and Child Mortality).* s.l.: National Statistical Office, Zomba, Malawi and ORC Macro Calverton, Maryland, USA, 2004. p. 123.

33. **WHO.** Health statistics and information systems. *World Health Organization.* [Online] 2017. http://www.who.int/healthinfo/statistics/indmaternalmortality/en/.

34. **PRI, Population Research Institute.** Definitions of maternal mortality. *www.pop.org.* [Online] https://www.pop.org/files/pub/doc/Maternal%20_Mortality_revised.pdf.

35. **WHO.** Health statistics and information systems-About the Global Burden of Disease (GBD) project. *World Health Organization.* [Online] 2017. http://www.who.int/healthinfo/global_burden_disease/about/en/.

36. Health statistics and information systems-Metrics: Disability-Adjusted Life Year (DALY. *World Health Organization.* [Online] 2017. http://www.who.int/healthinfo/global_burden_disease/metrics_daly/en/.

37. Quantifying environmental health impacts-Publications. *World Health Organization.* [Online] 2003. http://www.who.int/quantifying_ehimpacts/publications/en/9241546204chap3.pdf.

38. **Kahn, James G.** *UCSF-Philip R. Lee Institute for Health Policy Studies.* San Francisco, USA: s.n., 2014.

39. *QALYs vs DALYs vs LYs gained: What are the differences, and what difference do they make for health care priority setting?* **Robberstad, Bjarne.** 2, 2005, Norsk Epidemiologi, Vol. 15, pp. 183-191.

40. *Problems and solutions in calculating quality-adjusted life years (QALYs).* **Luis Prieto, José A Sacristán.** 80, 2003, Health and quality of life outcomes, Vol. 1.

41. **CDC.** Outbreak Case Definitions. *Centre for Disease Control and Prevention (CDC), Atlanta.* [Online] https://www.cdc.gov/urdo/downloads/casedefinitions.pdf.

42. Malaria (Plasmodium spp.) 2014 Case Definition. [Online] 2014. https://wwwn.cdc.gov/nndss/conditions/malaria/case-definition/2014/.

43. **WHO.** Global Malaria Program- WHO Malaria terminology. *WHO Malaria terminology.* s.l.: World Health Organization, 2016, pp. 9-11.

44. **NIMR.** *Guidelines for Diagnosis and Treatment of Malaria in India-2014.* New Delhi: NATIONAL VECTOR BORNE DISEASE CONTROL PROGRAMME, 2014. pp. 1-2.

45. **Silva, Isabel dos Santos.** *Cancer epidemiology: principles and methods.* Lyon: s.n., 1999. p. 190.

46. **BMJ.** Epidemiology for the uninitiated-Chapter 8. Case-control and cross-sectional studies. *The BMJ.* [Online] 2017. http://www.bmj.com/about-bmj/resources-readers/publications/epidemiology-uninitiated/8-case-control-and-cross-sectional.

47. **IIPS, International Institute for Population Sciences.** International Institute for Population Sciences, Mumbai, India. [Online] 2016. http://rchiips.org/NFHS/nfhs4.shtml.

48. **BMJ.** Epidemiology for the uninitiated- Chapter 7. Longitudinal studies. *The BMJ.* [Online] 2017. http://www.bmj.com/about-bmj/resources-readers/publications/epidemiology-uninitiated/7-longitudinal-studies.

49. *Study designs.* **Parab S, Bhalerao s.** 2, 2010, International journal of Ayurveda Research: (acessed through PMC), Vol. 1, p. PMC2924977. PMC2924977, 128–131. http://doi.org/10.4103/0974-7788.64406.

50. *Differences in Influenza Seasonality by Latitude, Northern India.* **Parvaiz A. Koul, Shobha Broor, Siddhartha Saha, John Barnes, Catherine Smith, Michael Shaw, Mandeep Chadha, and Renu B. Lal.** 10, 2014, Emerging Infectious Diseases Journal (CDC Atlanta), Vol. 20.

51. *Eradicating poliomyelitis: India's journey from hyperendemic to polio-free status.* **T. Jacob John, Vipin M. Vashishtha.** 2013, Indian J Med Res, pp. 881-894.

52. *Understanding the scientific basis of preventing polio by immunization. Pioneering contributions from India.* **TJ., John.** 2003. Proc Indian Natl Sci Acad. Vol. B69, pp. 393-422.

53. *Eradicating poliomyelitis: India's journey from hyperendemic to polio-free status.* **T Jacob John, Vipin M Vashishtha.** 5, 2013, Indian Journal of Medical Research., Vol. 137, pp. 881-894.

54. **World Bank.** Incidence of Tuberculosis: Global Tuberculosis Report by WHO. *The World Bank (https://data.worldbank.org).* [Online] 2015. https://data.worldbank.org/indicator/SH.TBS.INCD?type=shaded&view=map&year=2015.

55. **TBC-India.** TB India 2015, Revised National Tuberculosis Control Programme, Annual Status report, Central TB Division, Ministry of Health and Family Welfare, Govt of India. [Online] 2015. http://www.tbcindia.nic.in/showfile.php?lid=3166.

56. *Epidemic Investigation of the Jaundice Outbreak in Girdharnagar, Ahmedabad, Gujarat, India, 2008.* **Naresh T Chauhan, Prakash Prajapati, Atul V Trivedi, and A Bhagyalaxmi.** 2, 2010, Indian J Community Med, Vol. 35, pp. 294-297.

57. **WHO.** *Tuberculosis control in the South-East Asia Region.* s.l.: World Health Organization-Regional office for South-East Asia, 2015.

58. **WHO-SEAR.** *Tuberculosis control in the South-East Asia Region- Annual TB report 2015.* New Delhi: World Health Organization-Regional Office for South East Asia, 2015.

59. **NFHS-4.** International Istitute for Population Sciences. [Online] 2016. http://rchiips.org/NFHS/pdf/NFHS4/India.pdf.

60. *Epidemiology in Practice: Case-Control Studies (PMCID: PMC1706071).* **Susan Lewallen, MD and Paul Courtright, DrPH.** 28, 1998, Community Eye Health Journal, Vol. 11, pp. 57-58.

61. **UNC-SSW.** Public Health Social Work- Maternal and Child Health Leadership Training Program. *University of North Carolina at Chapel Hill.* [Online] https://ssw.unc.edu/mch/node/218.

62. **PSU.** Penn State University-Online course-Bias, Confoundingand Effect Modification STAT 507. *Penn State Eberly College of Science.* [Online] 2017. https://onlinecourses.science.psu.edu/stat507/node/34.

63. *Explaining Odds Ratios.* **Szumilas, Magdalena.** 3, 2010, J Can Acad Child Adolesc Psychiatry (PMCID: PMC2938757), Vol. 19, pp. 227-229.

64. *A Nationally Representative Case–Control Study of Smoking and Death in India.* **Prabhat Jha, M.D., Binu Jacob, M.Sc., Vendhan Gajalakshmi, Ph.D., Prakash**

C. Gupta, D.Sc., Neeraj Dhingra, M.D., Rajesh Kumar, M.D., Dhirendra N. Sinha, M.D., Rajesh P. Dikshit, Ph.D., Dillip K. Parida, M.D., Rajeev Kamadod, M.Sc., Jillian Boreham, Ph.D.,. 2008, The NEW ENGLAND JOURNAL of MEDICINE, Vol. 358, pp. 1137-1147.

65. *Effect of Duration of Exposure to Cement Dust on Respiratory Function of Non-Smoking Cement Mill Workers.* **Sultan Ayoub Meo, Abdul Majeed Al-Drees, Abeer A. Al Masri, Fawzia Al Rouq, and Muhammad Abdul Azeem.** 1, 2013, International Journal of Environmental Research and Public Health., Vol. 10, pp. 390-398.

66. **CPMC.** Coriel Personalized Medicine Collaborative. [Online] 2017. https://cpmc.coriell.org/genetic-education/understanding-risk.

67. *Understanding randomised controlled trials.* **Akobeng, A K.** s.l.: group.bmj.com, 2005, Arch Dis Child 2005;90:840–844. doi: 10.1136/adc.2004.058222(Downloaded from http://adc.bmj.com/on November 24, 2017), Vol. 90, p. 841.

68. *REVIEW ARTICLE-Randomized Controlled Trials.* **Maria Kabisch, Christian Ruckes, Monika Seibert-Grafe, Maria Blettner.** 2011, Deutsches Ärzteblatt International | Dtsch Arztebl Int 2011; 108(39): 663–8, pp. 663-668.

69. **Gray, Ronald.** Johns Hopkins Bloomberg School of Public Health-JHSPH OPEN courseware. *JHSPH OPEN courseware.* [Online] http://ocw.jhsph.edu/courses/Fundamentals Program Evaluation/PDFs/Lecture12.pdf.

70. **Howard White, Shagun Sabarwal and Thomas de Hoop.** Randomized Controlled Trials (RCTs)-Methodological Briefs, Impact Evaluation No.7. *http://www.unicef-irc.org/KM/IE/.* [Online] 2014. http://www.unicef-irc.org/KM/IE/.

71. **Pai, Madhukar.** Teach Epi-A website for learning and teaching epidemiology. [Online] http://www.teachepi.org/documents/courses/fundamentals/Pai_Lecture10_RCT.pdf.

72. **FDA, US.** U.S. Department of Food and Drug Administration-Department of Health and Human Services. [Online] 2017. https://www.fda.gov/For Patients/Approvals/Drugs/ucm405622.htm#phases.

73. *Observational and interventional study design types; an overview.* **Thiese, Matthew S.** 2, 2014, Biochem Med (Zagreb) v.24(2); 2014 Jun, Vol. 24, pp. 199-210.

74. **Priscilla Velengtas, Penny Mohr, Donna A. Messner.** Making Informed Decisions: Assessing the Strengths and Weaknesses of Study Designs and Analytic Methods for Comparative Effectiveness Research-A Briefing Document for Stakeholders. *National Pharmaceutical Council.* [Online] 2012. http://www.npcnow.org/publication/making-informed-decisions-assessing-strengths-and-weaknesses-study-designs-and-analytic.

75. **NIH.** Pub Med Health. *National Center for Biotechnology Information (NCBI) at the U.S. National Library of Medicine (NLM).* [Online] 2017. https://www.ncbi.nlm.nih.gov/pubmedhealth/PMHT0025849/.

76. **NIHR.** *Research Design Service, National Instituteof Health Research (NHS, UK).* [Online] http://www.rds-sc.nihr.ac.uk/study-design/quantitative-studies/clinical-trials/1017-2/.

77. *The n-of-1 clinical trial: the ultimate strategy for individualizing medicine? (Author manuscript).* **Elizabeth O Lillie, Bradley Patay, Joel Diamant, Brian Issell, Eric J Topol.** 2, 2011, Personalised Medicine. (retrievd from https://www.ncbi.nlm.nih.gov), Vol. 8, pp. 161-173.

78. *Fundamental deficiencies in the megatrial methodology.* **Charlton, Bruce G.** 1, s.l.: Bio Med Central, 2001, Available online http://cvm.controlled-trials.com/content/2/1/002 (retrieved from https://trialsjournal.biomedcentral.com/articles/10.1186/cvm-2-1-002), Vol. 2.

79. **SEFO.** DIFFERENT TYPES OF CLINICAL TRIALS. *Scientific European Federation of Osteopaths.* [Online] 2014. http://www.scientific-european-federation-osteopaths.org/different-types-of-clinical-trials/.

80. **Accord clinical Research.** Accord clinical Research,. [Online] 2017. https://www.accordclinical.com/clinical-study/types-of-clinical-trials/.

81. *Randomized Controlled Trials.* **Maria Kabisch, Christian Ruckes, Monika Seibert-Grafe, Maria Blettner.** 2011, Dtsch Arztebl Intv.108(39); 2011 Sep PMC3196997 (Retried from https://www.ncbi.nlm.nih.gov/pmc/articles/PMC3196997/).

82. *Blinding in clinical trials and other studies.* **Simon J Day, Douglas G Altman.** 7259, 2000, BMJ, Vol. 321, p. 504.

83. **CRD.** *Systematic Reviews-CRD's guidance for undertaking reviews in health care.* s.l.: CRD (Centre for Reviews and Dissemination), University of York, York Publishing Services Ltd, 2009. p. 11.

84. **NCI.** NCI Dictionary of Cancer Terms. *National Cancer Institute.* [Online] 2017. https://www.cancer.gov/publications/dictionaries/cancer-terms?cdrid=44160.

85. **Julian PT Higgins, Sally Green.** Some types of NRS design used for evaluating the effects of interventions. [book auth.] The Cochrane Collaboration. *Cochrane Handbook for Systematic Reviews of Interventions (online).* s.l.: The Cochrane Collaboration, 2011, Vol. Version 5.1.0, p. Table 13.1.a.

86. *Observational and interventional study design types; an overview.* **Thiese, Matthew S.** 2, 2014, Biochemia Medica, Vol. 24(, pp. 199-210.

87. *Evaluating non-randomised intervention studies.* **JJ Deeks, J Dinnes, R D'Amico, AJ Sowden, C Sakarovitch, F Song, M Petticrew, DG Altman.** 27, 2003, Health Technology Assessment, Vol. 7, p. 3.

88. **ADA.** Non-randomized trials: ADA Research Toolkit. [Online] 2011. https://www.researchgate.net/…non-randomized…/Non Randomized Trial.pdf.

89. *OVERVIEW OF RANDOMIZED CONTROLLED TRIALS- Review Article.* **Dr. Srikanth, Dr. Rathai Rajagopalan, Dr. Priyadarshini M.Deodurg,.** 3, 2013, Asian Journal of Pharmaceutical and Clinical Research, Vol. 6, pp. 32-38.

90. **Britton A, McKee M, Black N, McPherson K, Sanderson C, Bain C.** Choosing between randomised and non-randomised studies: a systematic review. *Health Technology Assessment.* 1998, Vol. 2, 13, pp. 21-22.

91. *The Choice of Controls for Providing Validity and Evidence in Clinical Research.* **Malay, S., & Chung, K. C.** 4, 2012, Vol. 130, pp. 959–965.

92. *Causation in epidemiology.* **M Parascandola, D L Weed.** 2011, J Epidemiol Community Health 2001;55:905–912 (retrieved from https://www.ncbi.nlm.nih.gov/pmc/articles/PMC1731812/pdf/v055p00905.pdf), Vol. 55, pp. 905-912.

93. **NHP.** Causation of Diseases. *National Health Portal, Govt. of India.* [Online] 2016. https://www.nhp.gov.in/causation-of-diseases_mtl.

94. **Gunther F. Craun, Rebecca L. Calderon.** HOW TO INTERPRET EPIDEMIOLOGICAL ASSOCIATIONS (Chapter 9). [book auth.] World Health Organization. *Nutrients in Drinking Water.* Genewa: World Health Organization, 2005, p. 113.

95. **Sukon Kanchanaraksa, PhD.** Causal Association. *JOHNS HOPKINS BLOOMBERG SCHOOL of PUBLIC HEALTH.* [Online] ocw.jhsph.edu/courses/Fund Epi II/PDFs/Lecture19.pdf.

96. *Public Health Classics-Association or causation: evaluating links between "environment and disease".* **Robyn M. Lucas, Anthony J. Mc Michael.** 10, 2005, Bulletin of the World Health Organization, Vol. 83, p. 793.

97. *Causal criteria in nutritional epidemiology.* **Nancy Potischman, Douglas L Weed.** 6, 1999, American Journal of Clinical Nutrition, Vol. 69, p. 1311S.

98. *The Environment and Disease: Association or Causation-President's Address.* **Hill, Sir A.B.** London: s.n., 1965. Proceedingsof the Royal Society of Medicine. Vol. 58.

99. **J. M. G. WILSON, G. JUNGNER.** *PRINCIPLES AND PRACTICE OF SCREENING (PUBLIC HEALTH PAPERS No-34).* Geneva: WHO, 1968.

100. *History of medical screening: from concepts to action.* **A Morabia, F F Zhang.** s.l.: BMJ, 2004, Postgrad Med J 2004;80:463–469. doi: 10.1136/pgmj.2004.018226, Vol. 80, pp. 463-469.

101. **J. M. G. WILSON, G. JUNGNER.** PUBLIC HEALTH PAPERS No. 34 PRINCIPLES AND PRACTICE OF SCREENING FOR DISEASE. Geneva: World Health Organization, 1968.

102. **CCI.** *Commission on Chronic Illness (1957), Chronic illnessin the United States; Volume I. Prevention of chronic illness, Cambridge, Mass, Harvard University Press. p 45, cited by JMG Wilson and G. Jungner in Public Health Paper No. 34, Principles of Screening.* 1957.

103. *Review article-Screening for Disease.* **Welch, William C. Black and H. Gilbert.** 1, 1997, American Journal of Roentgenology Diagnostic Imaging and Related Sciences (AJR:168, January 1997, Vol. 168, pp. 3-10.

104. *Understanding and using sensitivity, specificity and predictive values.* **Parikh, R., Mathai, A., Parikh, S., Chandra Sekhar, G., & Thomas, R.** 1, 2008, Indian Journal of Ophthalmology, 56(1), 45–50., Vol. 56, pp. 45-50.

105. **BU-SPH.** School of Public Health- Boston University. [Online] 2016. http://sphweb.bumc.bu.edu/otlt/mph-modules/ep/ep713_screening/ep713_screening5.html.

106. **Reingold, Arthur L.** Outbreak Investigations—A Perspective. *Emerging Infectious Diseases.* 1998, Vol. 4, 1, pp. 21-27.

107. **WHO.** Media Centre- Ebola virus disease fact sheet. *World Health Organization.* [Online] 2017. http://www.who.int/mediacentre/factsheets/fs103/en/.

108. **CDC.** *Self-Study Course SS1978Lesson 6-Centre for Disease Control and Prevention (CDC), Department of Health and Human Services, USA.* 2016.

109. **NHMRC.** Outbreak investigation and management guidelines. *National Healthand Medical Research Council-Australian Government.* [Online] 2010. https://www.nhmrc.gov.au/book/australian-guidelines-prevention-and-control-infection-healthcare-2010/b3-2-1-outbreak-investig.

110. **CDC.** *Centers for Disease Control and Prevention. Case definitions for infectious conditions under public health surveillance. MMWR Recommendations and Reports 1997:46 (RR-10):23-24.* Atlanta: CDC, 1997. pp. 23-24.

111. **IDSP.** INTEGRATED DISEASE SURVEILLANCE PROJECT- TRAINING MANUAL FOR STATE & DISTRICT SURVEILLANCE OFFICERS-CASE DEFINITIONS OF DISEASES & SYNDROMES UNDER SURVEILLANCE (Module 5). [book auth.] Integrated Disease Surveillance Project-Ministry of Health & Family Welfare. Government of India. p. 77.

112. **Merriam-Webster.** *Merriamm Webster Dictionary.* s.l.: Merriam-Webster Incorporate, 2018.
113. **Cambridge, Dictionary.** *Cambridge Dictionary (Online).* s.l.: CAMBRIDGE UNIVERSITY PRESS, 2018.
114. **WHO.** Health topics-Public health surveillance. *World Health organization.* [Online] 2017. http://www.who.int/topics/public_health_surveillance/en/.
115. **WHO-CDS.** Communicable disease surveillance and response: Guide to monitoring and evaluating. s.l.: World Health Organization, 2006.
116. **WHO.** Weekly Epidemiological Record (Volume 75; No. 1). *World Health Organization.* [Online] 2000. http://www.who.int/docstore/wer/pdf/2000/wer7501.pdf.
117. **CDC.** *MMWR-Centre for Disease Control and Prevention (CDC), Department of Health and Human Services, USA.* s.l.: Centre for Disease Control and Prevention (CDC), Department of Health and Human Services, USA, 1988. pp. 1-18.
118. Public Health 101 Series. *Centre for Disease Control and Prevention (CDC), Department of Health and Human Services, USA.* [Online] 2014. https://www.cdc.gov/publichealth101/documents/introduction-to-surveillance.pdf.
119. **Peter Nsubuga, Mark E. White, Stephen B. Thacker, Mark A. Anderson, Stephen B. Blount, Claire V. Broome, Tom M. Chiller, Victoria Espitia, Rubina Imtiaz, Dan Sosin, Donna F. Stroup, Robert V. Tauxe, Maya Vijayaraghavan, and Murray Trostle.** Public Health Surveillance: A Tool for Targeting and Monitoring Interventions. [book auth.] Breman JG, Measham AR, et al., editors In: Jamison DT. *Disease Control Priorities in Developing Countries. 2nd edition. Washington (DC): The International Bank for Reconstruction and Development/The World Bank; 2006. Chapter 53.* s.l.: Oxford University Press, 2006.
120. **WHO.** Laboratory training for field epidemiologists. *World Health Organization.* [Online] 2007. www.who.int/ihr/lyon/surveillance/lab_surveillance/ihr_l16surveillance_en.ppt.
121. **IDSP.** Integrated Disease Surveillance Programme, National Centre for Disease Control, Directorate General of Health Services, Ministry of Health and Family Welfare, Govt. of India. [Online] 2017. http://idsp.nic.in/.
122. **RL, Zimmern.** *Genetics in disease prevention. In: Puncheon D ed, Oxford handbook of public health practice.* Oxford: Oxford university press, 2001. pp. 544-549.
123. **Reingold, Arthur L.** Outbreak Investigations—A Perspective. *Emerging Infectious Diseases.* 1998, Vol. 4, 1, pp. 21-27.
124. **WHO.** Health statistics and information systems-About the Global Burden of Disease (GBD) projec. *World Health Organization.* [Online] 2017. http://www.who.int/healthinfo/global_burden_disease/about/en/.

125. World Health Organization-WHO Statistical Information System (WHOSIS). *WHO Statistical Information System (WHOSIS):*. [Online] 2006. http://www.who.int/whosis/whostat2006DefinitionsAndMetadata.pdf?ua=1.

126. **CDC.** *MMWR-Centre for Disease Control and Prevention (CDC), Department of Health and Human Services, USA.* s.l.: Centre for Disease Control and Prevention (CDC), Department of Health and Human Services, USA, 1988. pp. 1-18.

127. **BMJ.** Epidemiology for the uninitiated-Chapter 8. Case-control and cross sectional studies. *The BMJ.* [Online] 2017. http://www.bmj.com/about-bmj/resources-readers/publications/epidemiology-uninitiated/8-case-control-and-cross-sectional.

INDEX

A

Active Surveillance, 181
Allocation bias, 126
age specific mortality, 45
allocation bias, 126
attributable fraction, 110
Attributable Risk, 109

B

blinding, benefits of, 123
burden of disease, 51-53,

C

case-control studies, 92
case-fatality rate, 44
causal factors, strength of, 130
causal relation, establishing, 132
child mortality rate, 48
cohort studies, 104
Confounding, 94
consistency, of cuase, 132
continuous common-source
    epidemic, 168
critical point, 138
Cross Product Ratio, 102
cross-sectional studies, 72
crude death rate, 39

D

death to case ratio, 42
Descriptive epidemiological methods, 61
Disability Adjusted Life Years (DALYs), 52

E

Enabling factors, in causation, 131
Endemic, 27
Epidemic, 23
Epidemic, patterns, 24
Epidemic, investigations, 156
Epidemic, investigations team, 159-160
epidemic curve, 165
epidemiological methods, 61
epidemiological methods
    analytical, 62, 92
    descriptive, 61, 66
    experimental, 62, 114
    observational, 61, 92
etiological fraction, 110
exposure-disease association,
    analyzing, 98
external validity, 126

F

factorial trials, 120
factors in causation, 131

Index

G
generalizability, 126

H
Holoendemic, 28
Hyperendemic, 28
hypothesis, etiologic, 75
hypothesis, characteristics of, 76

I
incidence, 34
incidence, relation with prevalence, 38
infant mortality rate, 45-46
integrated surveillance, 183
internal validity, 126

L
Lead time, 139

M
matching, cases and controls, 94
maternal mortality rate, 49
maternal mortality ratio, 50
Mega trials, 127
mortality
    age specific, 45
    infant, 45
    maternal, 49
    measurement of, 39
    neonatal, 46
    post-neonatal, 47
    proportionate, 41
    sex-specific, 48
    under-five, 48

N
N-of-1 Trials, 120, 127
National Family Health Survey, 73
negative predictive value, 149
neonatal mortality rate, 46-47
Non-randomized controlled trials, 123

O
observational epidemiologic methods, 62
Odds ratio, 101
Open Trials, 122

P
pandemic, 28
passive surveillance, 180
period prevalence, 36
Person distribution, 86
personal characteristics, 5
Place distribution, 81
place patterns, 5
plausibility, 132
Population Attributable risk, 111
positive predictive value, 147
Post-neonatal mortality rate, 47
precipitating factors, 131
predisposing factors, 131
prevalence, 35
proportionate mortality, 41
prospective studies, 105

Q
Quality Adjusted Life Years (QALYs);, 56

R

Randomized controlled trials (RCT), 115
Relative Risk, 98, 107
Reinforcing factors, causation, 131
Reversibility, 133
Risk Difference, 110
Risk Ratio, 101

S

screening, 137
sensitivity, 143
sentinel surveillance, 181
Sequential Trials, 121
sex-specific mortality rate, 48
specificity, 144
sporadic, 28-29, 168
Strength of association, 133
surveillance, 174
surveillance, key characteristics of, 175
surveillance system, core functions, 178
surveillance, types, 180

T

temporal association, 132
Time distribution, 76, 78
time patterns, 4

Trials, crossover, 119
Trials, Efficacy vs. Effectiveness, 117
Trials, factorial, 120
Trials, Randomized Controlled, 115
Trials, Non-randomized, 115, 123
Trials, Superiority Vs. Equivalence Trials, 117
Trials, phase I, 117-118
Trials, phase II, 117-118
Trials, phase III, 117-118
Trials, phase IV, 118
Trials, Simple, two arm parallel, 118
Trials, N-of-1, 120
Trials, mega, 121
Trials, sequential, 121
Trials, open, 122
Trials, Single blind, 122
Trials, double blind, 122
Trials, triple blind, 122
Trials, quadruple blind, 122

U

under-five mortality rate, 48

W

wash-out period, 119

Made in the USA
Middletown, DE
28 April 2022

64848054R00128